Nontuberculous Mycobacteria

Editors

GWEN A. HUITT
CHARLES L. DALEY

CLINICS IN CHEST MEDICINE

www.chestmed.theclinics.com

March 2015 • Volume 36 • Number 1

ELSEVIER

1600 John F. Kennedy Boulevard • Suite 1800 • Philadelphia, Pennsylvania, 19103-2899

http://www.theclinics.com

CLINICS IN CHEST MEDICINE Volume 36, Number 1
March 2015 ISSN 0272-5231, ISBN-13: 978-0-323-35652-7

Editor: Patrick Manley
Developmental Editor: Casey Jackson

Clinics in Chest Medicine (ISSN 0272-5231) is published quarterly by Elsevier Inc., 360 Park Avenue South, New York, NY 10010-1710. Months of issue are March, June, September, and December. Periodicals postage paid at New York, NY and additional mailing offices. Subscription prices are $345.00 per year (domestic individuals), $556.00 per year (domestic institutions), $165.00 per year (domestic students/residents), $380.00 per year (Canadian individuals), $690.00 per year (Canadian institutions), $470.00 per year (international individuals), $690.00 per year (international institutions), and $230.00 per year (international and Canadian students/residents). International air speed delivery is included in all Clinics subscription prices. All prices are subject to change without notice. **POSTMASTER:** Send address changes to Clinics in Chest Medicine, Elsevier Health Sciences Division, Subscription Customer Service, 3251 Riverport Lane, Maryland Heights, MO 63043. **Customer Service: Telephone: 1-800-654-2452** (U.S. and Canada); **1-314-447-8871** (outside U.S. and Canada). **Fax: 1-314-447-8029. E-mail: journalscustomerservice-usa@elsevier.com (for print support); journalsonlinesupport-usa@elsevier.com (for online support).**

Reprints. For copies of 100 or more of articles in this publication, please contact the Commercial Reprints Department, Elsevier Inc., 360 Park Avenue South, New York, NY 10010-1710. Tel.: 212-633-3874; Fax: 212-633-3820; E-mail: reprints@elsevier.com.

Clinics in Chest Medicine is covered in *MEDLINE/PubMed (Index Medicus), Current Contents/Clinical Medicine, EMBASE/ Excerpta Medica, Science Citation Index,* and *ISI/BIOMED.*

Contributors

EDITORS

GWEN A. HUITT, MD, MS
Division of Mycobacterial and Respiratory Infections, National Jewish Health, Denver, Colorado

CHARLES L. DALEY, MD
Chief, Division of Mycobacterial and Respiratory Infections, National Jewish Health, Denver, Colorado

AUTHORS

EDWARD D. CHAN, MD
Division of Pulmonary Sciences and Critical Care Medicine, University of Colorado Denver Anschutz Medical Campus, Aurora, Colorado; Program in Cell Biology, Departments of Medicine and Academic Affairs, National Jewish Health; Denver Veterans Affairs Medical Center, Denver, Colorado

MARY ANN DE GROOTE, MD
Department of Microbiology, Immunology and Pathology, Colorado State University, Fort Collins, Colorado

ERIC F. EGELUND, PharmD, PhD
Infectious Disease Pharmacokinetics Laboratory, College of Pharmacy, Emerging Pathogens Institute, University of Florida, Gainesville, Florida

JOSEPH O. FALKINHAM III, PhD
Professor of Microbiology, Department of Biological Sciences, Virginia Tech, Blacksburg, Virginia

KEVIN P. FENNELLY, MD, MPH
College of Medicine, and Emerging Pathogens Institute, University of Florida, Gainesville, Florida

DAVID E. GRIFFITH, MD
Professor, Department of Medicine, University of Texas Health Science Center, Tyler, Texas

EMILY HENKLE, PhD, MPH
HIV, STD, and TB Section, Public Health Division, Oregon Health Authority, Portland, Oregon

JENNIFER R. HONDA, PhD
Division of Pulmonary Sciences and Critical Care Medicine, University of Colorado Denver Anschutz Medical Campus, Aurora, Colorado; Department of Medicine, National Jewish Health; Denver Veterans Affairs Medical Center, Denver, Colorado

SHANNON H. KASPERBAUER, MD
Division of Mycobacterial and Respiratory Infections, National Jewish Health, Denver, Colorado; Division of Infectious Diseases, University of Colorado Health Sciences Center, Aurora, Colorado

VIJAYA KNIGHT, MD, PhD
Department of Medicine, National Jewish Health, Denver, Colorado

THEODORE K. MARRAS, MD, MSc
Division of Respirology, Department of Medicine, University of Toronto and Toronto Western Hospital, Toronto, Ontario, Canada

STACEY L. MARTINIANO, MD
Assistant Professor, Department of Pediatrics, Children's Hospital Colorado, University of Colorado Denver School of Medicine, Aurora, Colorado

JOHN D. MITCHELL, MD
Courtenay C. and Lucy Patten Davis Endowed Chair in Thoracic Surgery; Professor and Chief, Section of General Thoracic Surgery, Division of Cardiothoracic Surgery, University of Colorado School of Medicine, Aurora, Colorado

JERRY A. NICK, MD
Professor, Department of Medicine, National Jewish Health, University of Colorado Denver, Denver, Colorado

CHARLES A. PELOQUIN, PharmD, FCCP
Professor and Director, Infectious Disease Pharmacokinetics Laboratory, College of Pharmacy, Emerging Pathogens Institute, University of Florida, Gainesville, Florida

JULIE V. PHILLEY, MD
Assistant Professor, Department of Medicine, University of Texas Health Science Center, Tyler, Texas

D. REBECCA PREVOTS, PhD, MPH
Epidemiology Unit, Laboratory of Clinical Infectious Diseases, Division of Intramural Research, National Institute of Allergy and Infectious Diseases, National Institutes of Health, Bethesda, Maryland

JAKKO VAN INGEN, MD, PhD
Department of Medical Microbiology, Radboud University Medical Center, Nijmegen, The Netherlands

KEVIN L. WINTHROP, MD, MPH
Division of Infectious Diseases; Division of Public Health and Preventative Medicine, Oregon Health and Science University, Portland, Oregon

Contents

Pulmonary disease is by far the most frequent disease caused by nontuberculous mycobacteria (NTM). To diagnose NTM pulmonary disease (NTM-PD), patients should have symptoms and radiologic signs suggestive of NTM-PD, and cultures of multiple respiratory tract samples must grow the same NTM species. Thus, the microbiological laboratory has a central role in the diagnosis of NTM-PD. This review summarizes currently available data on techniques involved in the microbiological diagnosis of NTM-PD, and aims to provide a framework for optimal microbiological diagnosis.

The treatment of infections caused by nontuberculous mycobacteria (NTM) is challenging because multidrug regimens with limited efficacy and considerable toxicity are required. Current treatment of NTM is largely empiric. None of the NTM drugs were specifically developed for the treatment of NTM; the rationale for their use was often extrapolated from the treatment of tuberculosis. This article reviews key features of the drugs that are most commonly used for NTM infections, and provides monitoring parameters. With this information, clinicians can make the most of the limited options available. Considerable research is needed to optimize the treatment of NTM.

Rapidly growing mycobacteria (RGM) include a diverse group of species. We address the treatment of the most commonly isolated RGM— *M abscessus* complex, *M fortuitum*, and *M chelonae*. The *M abscessus* complex is composed of 3 closely related species: *M abscessus* senso stricto (hereafter *M abscessus*), *M massiliense*, and *M bolletii*. Most studies address treatment of *M abscessus* complex, which accounts for 80% of lung disease caused by RGM and is the second most common RGM to cause extrapulmonary disease (after *M fortuitum*). The *M abscessus* complex represent the most drug-resistant nontuberculous mycobacteria and are the most difficult to treat.

The most common nontuberculous mycobacterial (NTM) lung pathogen, *Mycobacterium avium* complex (MAC), requires antibiotic treatment regimens that are long and often arduous. *M kansasii* is the slowly growing NTM pathogen with the most predictably successful treatment outcomes, whereas other slowly growing NTM pathogens such as *M xeonpi*, *M szulgai*, and *M malmoense* are less predictably responsive to antibiotic regimens. *M simiae* is the most difficult of the common slowly growing NTM pathogens to eradicate. Surgical intervention for slowly growing mycobacterial lung infection has proved beneficial for some patients, but the optimal candidates and timing for surgical intervention remain unknown.

Diseases and therapies that reduce cell-mediated immunity increase the risk of non-tuberculous mycobacterial (NTM) disease. Extrapulmonary NTM disease, including disseminated, skin, and catheter-related disease, is more common in immunosuppressed than immunocompetent patients. *Mycobacterium avium* complex remains the most common cause of NTM infection, but rapid growers including *Mycobacterium abscessus*, *Mycobacterium chelonae*, and *Mycobacterium fortuitum* play an important role in skin and catheter-related infections. With the exception of antibiotic prophylaxis for AIDS patients, the prevention of NTM remains difficult. Management is complicated, involving restoration of immune function and removal of catheters in addition to treatment with species-specific antibiotics per current guidelines.

Nontuberculous mycobacteria (NTM) are important emerging cystic fibrosis (CF) pathogens. Factors including the steady aging of the CF population, the apparent increase of NTM in the environment, and the potential for patient-to-patient transmission, may contribute to increased acquisition. Diagnosis of NTM disease is challenging due to disease overlap; thus, comprehensive care of the CF patient must be optimized to assess the clinical impact of the NTM (indolent versus active), and to improve response to treatment. The development of a CF-specific approach to the diagnosis and treatment of NTM infection is a research priority for the CF community.

The incidence of pulmonary nontuberculous mycobacterial disease is increasing. Despite aggressive medical therapy, a subset of patients will experience treatment failure or suffer disabling or life-threatening symptoms. The use of anatomic lung resection in addition to optimal medical management may, in select cases, result in improved clinical outcomes. More data are needed to confirm this approach. For those with nontuberculous mycobacterial infection, treatment in a multidisciplinary setting including surgeons familiar with operative techniques specific to infectious lung disease will improve patient care.

PROGRAM OBJECTIVE
The goal of the *Clinics in Chest Medicine* is to provide practitioners with state-of-the-art information that is clinically useful, concise, well referenced, and comprehensive.

TARGET AUDIENCE
All practicing physicians and healthcare professionals who provide patient care utilizing findings from *Chest Medicine Clinics of North America*.

LEARNING OBJECTIVES
Upon completion of this activity, participants will be able to:
1. Review the epidemiology of human pulmonary infection with non-tuberculous mycobacteria.
2. Discuss the treatment of rapidly and slow growing mycobacterial infections.
3. Recognize the approaches to non-tuberculous mycobacterial infections including medication and surgery.

ACCREDITATION
The Elsevier Office of Continuing Medical Education (EOCME) is accredited by the Accreditation Council for Continuing Medical Education (ACCME) to provide continuing medical education for physicians.

The EOCME designates this enduring material for a maximum of 15 *AMA PRA Category 1 Credit*(s)™. Physicians should claim only the credit commensurate with the extent of their participation in the activity.

All other health care professionals requesting continuing education credit for this enduring material will be issued a certificate of participation.

DISCLOSURE OF CONFLICTS OF INTEREST
The EOCME assesses conflict of interest with its instructors, faculty, planners, and other individuals who are in a position to control the content of CME activities. All relevant conflicts of interest that are identified are thoroughly vetted by EOCME for fair balance, scientific objectivity, and patient care recommendations. EOCME is committed to providing its learners with CME activities that promote improvements or quality in healthcare and not a specific proprietary business or a commercial interest.

The planning committee, staff, authors and editors listed below have identified no financial relationships or relationships to products or devices they or their spouse/life partner have with commercial interest related to the content of this CME activity:
Edward D. Chan, MD; Eric F. Egelund, PharmD, PhD; Joseph O. Falkinham, III, PhD; David E. Griffith, MD, FACP, FCCP; Kristen Helm; Emily Henkle, PhD, MPH; Jennifer R. Honda, PhD; Brynne Hunter; Shannon H. Kasperbauer, MD; Vijaya Knight, MD, PhD; Sandy Lavery; Patrick Manley; Theodore K. Marras, MD, MSc; Stacey L. Martiniano, MD; John D. Mitchell, MD; Palani Murugesan; Jerry A. Nick, MD; Charles A. Peloquin, PharmD, FCCP; D. Rebecca Prevots, PhD, MPH; Jakko van Ingen, MD, PhD.

The planning committee, staff, authors and editors listed below have identified financial relationships or relationships to products or devices they or their spouse/life partner have with commercial interest related to the content of this CME activity:
Charles L. Daley, MD has a research grant from Insmed.
Mary Ann De Groote, MD is a consultant/advisor for SomaLogic, Inc.; spouse has an employment affiliation with, and has royalties/patents with SomaLogic, Inc.; has a research grant from Crestone, Inc.; spouse/partner is a consultant/advisor for and has royalties/patents with Crestone, Inc.
Kevin P. Fennelly, MD, MPH is a consultant/advisor for InsMed.
Gwen A. Huitt, MD, MS is a consultant/advisor for The Phoenix Group.
Julie V. Philley, MD is a consultant/advisor for Insmed.
Kevin L. Winthrop, MD, MPH has a research grant from Insmed.

UNAPPROVED/OFF-LABEL USE DISCLOSURE
The EOCME requires CME faculty to disclose to the participants:
1. When products or procedures being discussed are off-label, unlabelled, experimental, and/or investigational (not US Food and Drug Administration (FDA) approved); and
2. Any limitations on the information presented, such as data that are preliminary or that represent ongoing research, interim analyses, and/or unsupported opinions. Faculty may discuss information about pharmaceutical agents that is outside of FDA-approved labelling. This information is intended solely for CME and is not intended to promote off-label use of these medications. If you have any questions, contact the medical affairs department of the manufacturer for the most recent prescribing information.

TO ENROLL
To enroll in the *Chest Medicine Clinics* Continuing Medical Education program, call customer service at 1-800-654-2452 or sign up online at http://www.theclinics.com/home/cme. The CME program is available to subscribers for an additional annual fee of USD $225.

METHOD OF PARTICIPATION

In order to claim credit, participants must complete the following:

1. Complete enrolment as indicated above.
2. Read the activity.
3. Complete the CME Test and Evaluation. Participants must achieve a score of 70% on the test. All CME Tests and Evaluations must be completed online.

CME INQUIRIES/SPECIAL NEEDS

For all CME inquiries or special needs, please contact elsevierCME@elsevier.com.

CLINICS IN CHEST MEDICINE

RELATED INTEREST

Clinics in Laboratory Medicine, Vol. 34, No. 2 (June 2014)
Respiratory Infections
Michael J. Loeffelholz, *Editor*

DOWNLOAD Free App!

Review Articles
THE CLINICS

NOW AVAILABLE FOR YOUR iPhone and iPad

Preface
Nontuberculous Mycobacteria

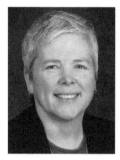 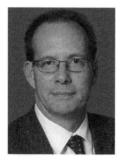

Gwen A. Huitt, MD, MS   Charles L. Daley, MD
Editors

Nontuberculous mycobacteria (NTM) represent over 160 separate species that vary greatly in their ability to cause disease in humans. Epidemiologic data from across the world have documented increasing prevalence of pulmonary NTM infections and, in some areas, prevalence rates are greater than those of tuberculosis. This issue is dedicated to NTM and reviews the pathogenesis, epidemiology, diagnosis, and management of these complex and difficult-to-treat infections. The issue begins with a review of the pathogenesis of NTM infections, highlighting the spectrum of host impairment associated with NTM disease. An extensive review of the epidemiology of NTM infections follows. This article delineates the varying rates of disease and increasing prevalence of NTM pulmonary disease globally. Possible reasons for the increasing prevalence are explored, including exposure to environmental sources and possible steps that can be taken to decrease exposure.

Diagnosis of pulmonary NTM infections requires that the clinician integrate clinical, radiographic, and microbiological data but, ultimately, the diagnosis is based on isolation of the organism from the patient. The laboratory diagnosis of NTM is in a state of evolution, transitioning from mostly phenotypic to molecular methods. The next article summarizes available data on techniques for the microbiological diagnosis of NTM pulmonary disease and provides a framework for the optimal microbiological diagnosis.

The first article to address treatment reviews the commonly used drugs for the treatment of NTM infections and approach to monitoring for adverse reactions. The drugs and regimens used will vary depending on the species causing disease. Therefore, treatment is discussed by dividing the reviews into one that reviews the management of rapidly growing mycobacteria and another for slowly growing mycobacteria. NTM infections are increasingly common in some special populations, so we have included reviews of the management of NTM infections in immunocompromised patients and persons with cystic fibrosis. And, finally, in some cases, antimicrobial therapy is insufficient for control and/or cure of the infection. In these cases, surgical resection may be indicated, so we have included an excellent review of the surgical approach to pulmonary NTM infections.

We hope this issue is of interest to clinicians, scientists, and patients. To the authors, we owe them thanks for their excellent contributions. To Casey Jackson and the Elsevier staff, we thank you for your support and patience during the long effort to bring this issue to fruition and now publication.

Clin Chest Med 36 (2015) xi–xii
http://dx.doi.org/10.1016/j.ccm.2014.11.006
0272-5231/15/$ – see front matter © 2015 Published by Elsevier Inc.

We would like to dedicate this issue to the memory of Fern Leitman, a patient, visionary, and leader in the fight against NTM.

Gwen A. Huitt, MD, MS
Division of Mycobacterial and
Respiratory Infections
National Jewish Health
1400 Jackson Street
Denver, CO 80206, USA

Charles L. Daley, MD
Division of Mycobacterial and
Respiratory Infections
National Jewish Health, Room J304
1400 Jackson Street
Denver, CO 80206, USA

E-mail addresses:
huittg@njhealth.org (G.A. Huitt)
daleyc@njhealth.org (C.L. Daley)

Erratum

An error was made in the December 2014 issue (Volume 35, Number 4) of *Clinics in Chest Medicine* on page 793 of the article "Steroids for Acute Respiratory Distress Syndrome?" regarding the incorrect listing of references 28 and 29. The correct references are as follows:

28. Festic E, Ortiz-Diaz E, Lee A, et al. United States Critical Illness and Injury Trials Group: Lung Injury Prevention Study Investigators (USCIITG-LIPS). Prehospital use of inhaled steroids and incidence of acute lung injury among patients at risk. J Crit Care 2013;28(6):985–91.

29. Karnatovskaia LV, Lee AS, Gajic O, et al. U.S. Critical Illness and Injury Trials Group: Lung Injury Prevention Study Investigators (USCIITG-LIPS). The influence of prehospital systemic corticosteroid use on development of acute respiratory distress syndrome and hospital outcomes. Crit Care Med 2013;41(7): 1679–85.

Clin Chest Med 36 (2015) xiii
http://dx.doi.org/10.1016/j.ccm.2014.12.001
0272-5231/15/$ – see front matter © 2015 Elsevier Inc. All rights reserved.

Pathogenesis and Risk Factors for Nontuberculous Mycobacterial Lung Disease

Jennifer R. Honda, PhD[a,b,c], Vijaya Knight, MD, PhD[b],
Edward D. Chan, MD[a,b,c],*

KEYWORDS

- Nontuberculous mycobacteria • Lung disease • Risk factors • Pathogenesis

KEY POINTS

- Nontuberculous mycobacteria (NTM) are ubiquitous in the environment, and yet NTM lung disease is relatively uncommon and is dominated by relatively few species of NTM.
- These observations suggest that both host vulnerability and pathogen virulence factors are important determinants of whether infections become established.
- There are risk factors for isolated NTM lung disease and disseminated disease as well as components of NTM cell envelope that are likely to play important pathogenic roles.

INTRODUCTION

Nontuberculous mycobacteria (NTM) infections can be broadly classified as skin and soft tissue infections, isolated lung disease, and visceral or disseminated disease. The importance of this nosologic distinction is that the degree of underlying immune abnormalities varies between each of them. At one end of the spectrum, skin and soft tissue infections are almost always the result of iatrogenic or accidental inoculation of NTM caused by surgical contamination, trauma, and so forth in otherwise normal hosts. Patients with NTM lung disease not uncommonly have a primary lung disorder or a systemic condition that predisposes them to these infections. At the other end of the spectrum, visceral and disseminated NTM disease invariably occurs in individuals with more severe immunosuppression. Although the focus of this article is to discuss the pathogenesis of NTM lung disease, the authors also briefly summarize the risk factors of visceral/disseminated NTM disease as they provide insights into host-defense mechanisms against these organisms.

KNOWN RISK FACTORS FOR NONTUBERCULOUS MYCOBACTERIA LUNG DISEASE

NTM lung disease occurs primarily in 3 broad groups of patients (**Fig. 1**): (1) those with anatomic lung abnormalities that usually do not have an identifiable genetic basis (eg, localized bronchiectasis from prior unrelated infections, emphysema, and pneumoconiosis, such as silicosis),[1–3] (2) those with immunologic or known or suspected

Disclosures: none.
[a] Division of Pulmonary Sciences and Critical Care Medicine, University of Colorado Denver Anschutz Medical Campus, Aurora, CO 80045, USA; [b] Program in Cell Biology, Department of Medicine, National Jewish Health, Denver, CO 80206, USA; [c] Denver Veterans Affairs Medical Center, Denver, CO 80220, USA
* Corresponding author. National Jewish Health, D509, Neustadt Building, 1400 Jackson Street, Denver, CO 80206.
E-mail address: chane@njhealth.org

Clin Chest Med 36 (2015) 1–11
http://dx.doi.org/10.1016/j.ccm.2014.10.001
0272-5231/15/$ – see front matter Published by Elsevier Inc.

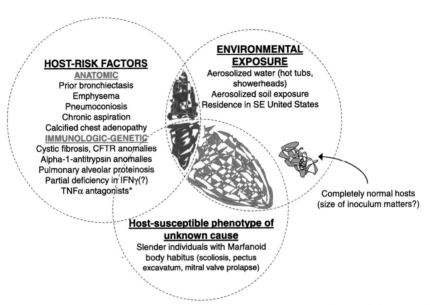

Fig. 1. Venn diagram of the risk factors for NTM lung disease. The intersection of host risk factors and significant environmental exposure to NTM are likely requirements for establishment of disease. * Can result in either isolated lung disease or disseminated disease. CFTR, cystic fibrosis transmembrane conductance regulator; IFNγ, interferon-gamma; SE, Southeastern; TNFα, tumor necrosis factor-alpha.

genetic disorders that predispose to bronchiectasis and/or lung infections (eg, cystic fibrosis, primary ciliary dyskinesia, alpha-1-antitrypsin deficiency, Williams-Campbell syndrome, Mounier-Kuhn syndrome, Sjögren syndrome, pulmonary alveolar proteinosis, and common variable immunodeficiency),[4–8] and (3) those with no known overt lung or immunologic abnormalities.[9–11] The pathophysiologic mechanisms by which immunologic and/or genetic disorders predispose to isolated NTM lung disease are listed in **Table 1**.

NONTUBERCULOUS MYCOBACTERIA LUNG DISEASE IN PATIENTS WITHOUT A KNOWN UNDERLYING CAUSE

The occurrence of NTM lung disease in individuals without any known predisposing condition is well known; it has been observed that not an insignificant number of these patients possess a lifelong slender body habitus and thoracic cage abnormalities, such as pectus excavatum and scoliosis.[10,12–15]

A plausible mechanism by which slender individuals with low body fat content may be predisposed to NTM infections is relative deficiency of leptin, an adipokine whose canonical function is that of a satiety hormone. However, leptin has several immunomodulatory functions that can potentially enhance host immunity against NTM, including the differentiation of uncommitted T_0

cells toward the T_H1 interferon-gamma (IFNγ)-producing phenotype.[16] Indeed, leptin-deficient mice are more susceptible to *Mycobacterium abscessus* experimental lung infection.[17] Patients

Table 1
Major known mechanisms that predispose to primary or secondary NTM lung disease

Mechanism for Predisposition	Associated Conditions
Primary or ciliary dysfunction	Primary ciliary dyskinesia, bronchiectasis of any cause
Inspissated secretions	Cystic fibrosis
Structural lung disease	Emphysema, bronchiectasis of any cause
Macrophage dysfunction	Alpha-1-antitrypsin deficiency or anomaly, silica exposure, pulmonary alveolar proteinosis
Deficiency of specific immune molecules	Antitumor necrosis factor-alpha therapy, common variable immunodeficiency
Cartilage deficiency in airways	Williams-Campbell syndrome
Elastin deficiency in airways	Mounier-Kuhn syndrome

with pulmonary NTM have been found to have reduced serum leptin levels[15] or a loss in the normal direct relationship between serum leptin concentration and percent body fat.[18]

The aforementioned thoracic cage abnormalities described in patients with pulmonary NTM are some of the features of Marfan syndrome (MFS), a genetic disorder caused by mutations of the FIBRILLIN-1 gene. Although most of the patients with pulmonary NTM do not manifest classic MFS, some FIBRILLIN-1 mutations may display a mild or subclinical variant of MFS.[19] A pathophysiologic mechanism that helps support this hypothesis is that the connective tissue defect seen with MFS is considered to be caused by increased localized production of transforming growth factor-beta (TGFβ), a cytokine known to predispose to NTM infection.[19–21] In light of this, patients with NTM have been found to have increased TGFβ and decreased IFNγ production compared with controls.[18] NTM lung disease was reported in a patient with congenital contractural arachnodactyly, a genetic disorder caused by FIBRILLIN-2 gene mutation that shares many clinical features with MFS.[22] If indeed the MFS-NTM hypothesis is true, it must be explained why some case series of patients with pulmonary NTM show a predominance of postmenopausal women because the FIBRILLIN-1 gene is located on chromosome 15; therefore, any mutations would be expected to affect both sexes equally. Possibilities include (1) declining estrogen levels with aging provide a permissive role if one already possesses a susceptibility factor because estrogen is protective against NTM infection in mice[23]; (2) referral bias of women; and/or (3) the unproven notion that women are less inclined to expectorate effectively than men, preventing them from clearing their infections, the so-called Lady Windermere syndrome. Indeed, in a study of 6 families with clustering of pulmonary NTM disease, 31% of whom had scoliosis, most of the affected individuals were women despite the fact that the patterns of transmission were consistent with dominant and recessive modes of inheritance.[24] Fowler and coworkers[25] have also described reduced ciliary beat frequency in the nasal epithelium of patients with pulmonary NTM compared with controls.[25]

KNOWN RISK FACTORS FOR VISCERAL OR DISSEMINATED NONTUBERCULOUS MYCOBACTERIA DISEASE

Patients with visceral or disseminated NTM disease are almost always frankly immunocompromised, such as those receiving tumor necrosis factor-alpha (TNFα) antagonists, organ transplant recipients, and patients with untreated AIDS (**Table 2**). Although rare, certain inherited disorders can also predispose to NTM and are termed mendelian susceptibility to mycobacterial diseases (MSMD) (see **Table 2**). These experiments-of-nature provide great insights into which elements of the immune system are host protective against mycobacteria. Although some MSMD have not been reported to be associated with NTM infections, they are found to be risk factors for disseminated infection with bacilli Calmette-Guérin (BCG), a minimally pathogenic mycobacteria; thus, a lack of NTM-associated disease with some MSMD may simply be caused by happenstance or the failure to recognize the presence of an underlying disorder.

PATHOGENESIS OF CENTRILOBULAR NODULES, BRONCHIECTASIS, AND CAVITIES IN NONTUBERCULOUS MYCOBACTERIA LUNG DISEASE

The hallmark radiographic features of NTM lung disease include bronchiectasis, nodules, tree-in-bud opacities (branching centrilobular nodules) with and without cavities, atelectasis, ground-glass opacities, and/or consolidation. Correlation of these radiographic features with histopathology can help elucidate the cellular pathogenesis of NTM lung disease, independent of any underlying predisposing condition.[26–28] In resected lung tissues, computed tomography findings of bronchiectasis and bronchiolitis correlated with peribronchial and peribronchiolar granulomatous inflammation as well as airway wall necrosis.[26] Lung nodules and cavity walls were also found to be composed of caseating granulomas; the outer rim of cavity walls may be surrounded by myofibroblasts, the differentiation of which requires the immunosuppressive cytokine TGFβ.[26]

Clinical experience indicates that NTM can exacerbate preexisting bronchiectasis but can also cause de novo bronchiectasis. Supporting evidence for the latter is the finding that NTM-associated nodules and air-space disease may precede the development of bronchiectasis. Based on histopathologic correlations, bronchiectasis may develop by at least 2 distinct but similar mechanisms (**Fig. 2**). One mechanism is a weakened airway wall caused by chronic granulomatous inflammation leading to mucosal ulceration and atrophy. Another mechanism is bronchial and bronchiolar dilatation caused by airway obstruction by chronic inflammatory mucous plugs. It has also been speculated, based partly on the presence of a patent, feeding bronchus

Table 2
Known predisposing conditions to visceral or disseminated NTM disease

Gene	Mode of Inheritance	Underlying Pathogenic Disorder	Comments	Reference
N/A	N/A	Use of TNFα antagonists, block TNFα-mediated immune responses, such as phagolysosomal maturation, monocyte apoptosis, and IFNγ production	Can predispose to either isolated lung or extrapulmonary disease	Winthrop et al,[56] 2013
N/A	N/A	Immunosuppression seen in organ transplant recipients	Skin, pulmonary, and catheter-related infections	Doucette et al,[57] 2004
N/A	N/A	Patients with untreated AIDS resulting in CD4$^+$ T cell depletion, impaired cytolytic CD8$^+$ T-cell activation, and inadequate killing of mycobacteria by macrophages	Increased susceptibility to disseminated NTM infections and *M kansasii* associated lung disease.	French et al,[58] 1997
IFNγR1 (ligand binding chain of IFNγR)	AD, AR	Impaired cellular responses to IFNγ	Extreme susceptibility to disseminated NTM infections	Dorman et al,[59] 2004
IFNγR2 (signal transducing chain of IFNγR)	AR	Impaired cellular responses to IFNγ	Same as above	Döffinger et al,[60] 2000
STAT1α	AD	Impaired cellular response to IFNγ and IFNα/β	Increased susceptibility to mycobacterial and viral infections	Dupuis et al,[61] 2001
IL-12 p40 subunit	AR	Lack of IL-12 production leading to defective activation and differentiation of T_H1 cells	Milder phenotype with broader susceptibility to intracellular infections (salmonella, mycobacteria, Nocardia, fungi and Leishmania)	Prando et al,[62] 2013
IL-12 receptor β1 subunit	AR	Defective IL-12 signaling resulting in suboptimal activation and differentiation of T_H1 cells	Same as above	Haverkamp et al,[63] 2014
Tyrosine kinase 2 (TYK2)	AR	Impaired response to IL-12, IFNαβ, and IL-10	Generalized infection with low virulence mycobacteria (BCG); increased susceptibility to viral and fungal infections	Minegishi et al,[64] 2006

(continued on next page)

Table 2
(continued)

Gene	Mode of Inheritance	Underlying Pathogenic Disorder	Comments	Reference
NF-κB essential modulating factor (NEMO/ IKBKG)	X-linked	Selective impairment of IL-12 production in monocytes and dendritic cells, partially attributed to impairment of CD40L-IL-12 pathway	Increased susceptibility to M tuberculosis and BCG with intact immunity to pyogenic infections	Filipe-Santos et al,[65] 2006
N/A	N/A	Acquired autoantibodies to IFNγ (HLA linkage)	Increased susceptibility to extrapulmonary and disseminated NTM infections	Chi et al,[66] 2013
MonoMAC syndrome (mutations in GATA binding protein 2)	AD and sporadic	Profound monocytopenia and NK- and B-cell lymphocytopenia Frequent CD4+ and CD8+ lymphocytopenia	Myelodysplasia, pulmonary alveolar proteinosis, disseminated NTM and human papilloma virus infections; increased susceptibility to opportunistic fungi	Hsu et al,[67] 2013
Cytochrome b-245, β polypeptide (CYBB)	X-linked	Selective defect in monocyte-derived macrophage oxidative burst	Disseminated M tuberculosis or BCG infection	Bustamante et al,[68] 2011
Interferon stimulated gene 15 (ISG15)	AR	Decreased production of IFNγ by T and NK cells	Milder mycobacterial infections, similar to IL-12 defects	Bogunovic et al,[69] 2012
Interferon regulatory factor 8 (IRF8)	AD, AR	Inadequate priming of T cells to produce IFNγ	Milder course of infection, recurrent episodes of disseminated BCG-disease	Hambleton et al,[70] 2011

Abbreviations: AD, autosomal dominant; AR, autosomal recessive; BCG, bacilli Calmette-Guérin; IFNγR1, interferon-gamma receptor 1; IL, interleukin; N/A, not-applicable; NEMO/IKBKG, nuclear factor-kappa-B essential modulator/inhibitor of NFkappaB kinase subunit gamma; NF-κB, nuclear factor kappaB; NK, natural killer; STAT1alpha, signal transducer and activator of transcription 1.

leading to the cavity, that some NTM cavities are formed from progressive cystic dilatation of bronchi.[27]

What are some plausible molecular and cellular mechanisms by which NTM infection ultimately leads to bronchiectasis? The inability to eradicate NTM in the lungs, whether caused by an underlying predisposing condition and/or infection with a large inoculum that overwhelms the host immune response, can result in the recruitment of an exuberant inflammatory response, orchestrated by immune and airway epithelial cells through the release of inflammatory cytokines and chemokines. Recruited neutrophils can cause damage to the airway epithelium through the release of elastase and metalloproteinases, proteolytic enzymes that can erode mucosal barriers resulting in NTM-containing microabscesses. Elastase may also cause ciliary dysfunction, mucous gland hyperplasia, and mucus hypersecretion that further impairs clearance and may enhance M abscessus biofilm formation.[29,30] Moreover, elastase and other proteases cleave Fcγ receptors and complement receptor 1 from neutrophil surfaces as well as digest immunoglobulins and complement components from mycobacterial surfaces. These activities impair opsonization of mycobacteria and reduce their recognition by neutrophils, leading to decreased phagocytosis and bacterial killing.[29] Elastase can also inhibit efferocytosis, a process whereby apoptotic neutrophils are phagocytosed.[29] As a result, dead neutrophils can incite

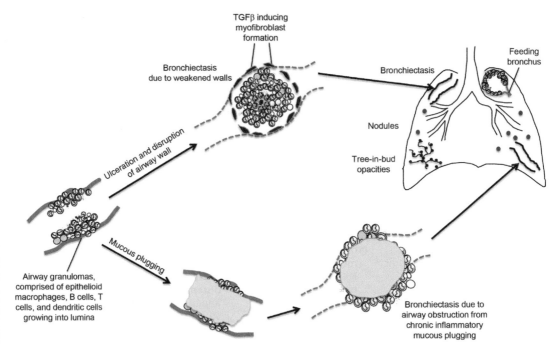

Fig. 2. Histopathologic-radiographic correlation of NTM lung disease. The key histopathologic finding in NTM lung disease is airway wall granuloma that may manifest radiographically as tree-in-bud pattern and nodules. The mechanisms of airway dilatation, bronchiolectasis and bronchiectasis, include disruption and weakening of the airway wall caused by chronic inflammation and actions of various proteolytic enzymes as well as chronic inflammatory airway obstruction caused by mucous plugging.

further inflammation and release highly viscous DNA that contributes to the volume and inspissated quality of bronchiectatic mucous.

PATHOGENESIS OF NONTUBERCULOUS MYCOBACTERIA INFECTION OF HOST CELLS

Given the airway-centric nature of NTM infection in the lungs, it is not surprising that NTM can infect bronchial epithelial cells. Fibronectin-attachment protein is present on the surface of M avium and, by binding to fibronectin on mucosal surfaces, serves to facilitate more specific mycobacterial binding to integrin receptors.[31] Bacilli that have gained entry into epithelial cells undergo a phenotypic change that results in greater efficiency at invading macrophages.[31] Biofilm formation and NTM-mediated inhibition of inflammatory cytokine production are mechanisms that can subvert host immunity and promote colonization and subsequent invasion of the bronchial epithelium.[31]

NTM opsonized with complement components, such as C3b and C4b, are also able to gain entry into alveolar macrophages following binding to complement receptors present on the phagocytes; other macrophage receptors involved in phagocytosis of NTM include mannose receptors and scavenger receptors.[31] The multiple pathways by which NTM are able to enter macrophages suggest that the intracellular niche is a favorable adaptation for the bacilli if the phagocytes are not primed to kill the bacteria. Immune-evasion mechanisms by which NTM are able to survive within macrophages include inhibition of phagosome-lysosome fusion, shift in metabolism to a more anaerobic intracellular environment, induction of NTM-related genes that enhance replication, direct inhibition of host macrophage function and lymphocyte proliferation, and possibly through induction of macrophage apoptosis.[31,32]

VIRULENCE MECHANISMS OF NONTUBERCULOUS MYCOBACTERIA
Lipids of Nontuberculous Mycobacteria

NTM-specific virulence factors likely help drive the establishment and progression of disease (**Fig. 3**). This notion is supported by the fact that, even though more than 160 species of NTM are identified, most diseases are caused by relatively few species. The most widely recognized virulence factor of the *Mycobacterium* genus is its waxy cell envelope that protects against antibiotics and host immune defenses as well as facilitates survival in soil and water. Lipids of various composition compose up to 60% of the mycobacterial cell envelope compared with 20% in gramnegative bacteria.[33] There are at least 4 major groups of lipids represented in the NTM envelope: phospholipids, apolar lipids, amphipathic lipids, and glycolipids.

NTM-derived lipids contribute to pathogenesis by subverting the host immune responses. Total lipid extracts from *M avium* suppressed the production of IFNγ and TNFα, cytokines important in controlling NTM infections.[34] Moreover, incubation of human peripheral blood mononuclear cells (PBMC) with total lipids from *M avium* increased both the secretion of immunosuppressive molecules, such as prostaglandin E_2, by macrophages and the replication of intracellular NTM.[35] These findings indicate that NTM lipids can suppress T_H1 and increase T_H2 immune responses. Although in toto NTM-derived lipids can modulate immune responses that result in enhanced survival of the bacilli, the ability of glycopeptidolipids (GPL) and lipoglycans to function as virulence factors is discussed later.

Glycopeptidolipids

The GPL are produced solely by NTM organisms and are absent from *M tuberculosis* and *M leprae*.[36] For *M smegmatis*, nearly 85% of all surface lipids are GPL; this percentage is likely to be higher or lower depending on the serovar and species of NTM. There are 2 main classes of GPL, both of which are noncovalently bound to the cell envelope's outer most layer. The first class is the apolar, nonspecific GPL (nsGPL) produced by many NTM, particularly *M abscessus*. At a minimum, nsGPL consist of a tripeptide-amino alcohol core with an amide-linked long-chain fatty acid. The second class, commonly produced by *M avium*, includes a variety of polar, serovarspecific GPL (ssGPL) that show sufficient antigenicity to be used as potential serodiagnostic markers.[37] The ssGPL consist of various oligosaccharides attached onto the tetrapeptide core of nsGPL. There are approximately 31 different ssGPL that have been identified, but their in vivo biological activities remain ill defined. Nonetheless, GPL are one of the most multifunctional lipids of NTM.

Although NTM do not possess flagella, pili, or fimbriae, they are able to slide on surfaces of culture medium. GPL are essential for both the sliding phenotype and biofilm formation by NTM.[38,39] Therefore, it seems plausible to think that NTM capable of a sliding movement and forming biofilms will likely be better colonizers of the respiratory mucosa.

The composition and concentration of GPL vary per species and can impact colony morphology. *M abscessus* containing nsGPL show a smooth morphotype; those lacking nsGPL because of small genetic interruptions in the mycobacterial peptide synthetase locus manifest as rough morphotypes.[40] *M abscessus* smooth variants survive in the environment, are noninvasive, and initiate infection in susceptible hosts. To deter recognition by toll-like receptor 2 (TLR2) present on innate immune cells, GPL of smooth *M abscessus* form an outer layer that covers the mycobacterial TLR2 ligand phosphatidyl-myo-inositol mannosides, effectively cloaking the glycolipid from being recognized by TLR2.[41] For reasons not well characterized, the more virulent, rough morphotype emerges later, sometimes several years after the initial infection.[42] In a murine model, Byrd and Lyons[40] demonstrated that human monocytes eradicated infection by smooth *M abscessus*, whereas rough variants persisted and propagated in the intracellular phagosome.[40] Clinical and epidemiologic data also associate rough variants with more severe and persistent pulmonary disease.[43] The triggers for *M abscessus* morphotype switching in vivo remain unknown. However, based on whole-genome analyses, switching between forms is likely an infrequent occurrence.[44] *M avium* also produces smooth and rough variants; but unlike *M abscessus*, the transition between forms is irreversible and caused by the loss of genes involved in GPL biosynthesis.[45]

Although the absence of nsGPL from *M abscessus* facilitates intracellular survival, *M avium* ssGPL are required for intracellular survival and impact cytokine responses, suggesting serovar oligosaccharides contribute to species-specific pathogenesis.[46] The immunomodulatory activities of *M avium* ssGPL are varied and depend on the serovar from which they were extracted (eg, ssGPL from *M avium* serovar 1, 2, and 8, which are different enough from the ssGPL of serovars 4 or 20, induce the production of TNFα and/ or prostaglandin E_2 by human PBMC).[46,47] ssGPL also promote phagocytosis and inhibit phagosome-lysosome fusion.[48] Because GPL resist degradation by lysosomal enzymes, accumulate inside host macrophages, and are shed in exosomes, they can potentially trigger neighboring macrophages.[49,50]

Allelic exchange mutagenesis and the ts-sacB (thermosensitive sucrose utilization enzyme) selection system have been used to create ssGPL null mutants from wild-type *M avium* serovars 2 and 8 for genetic studies. A study with these variants showed that serovar 2 ssGPL facilitated invasion of macrophages, suppressed TNFα

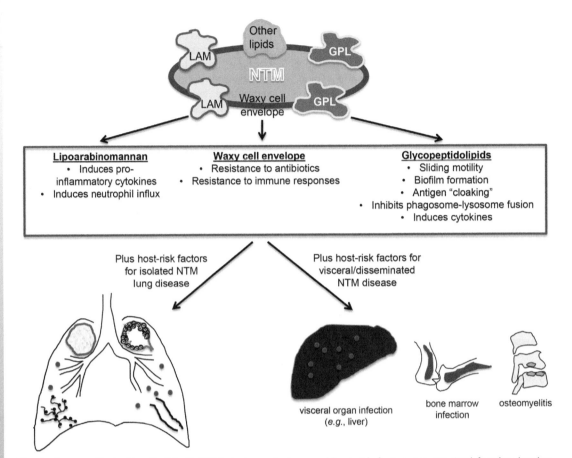

Fig. 3. Cartoon illustrating that both NTM virulence factors and host-risk factors are required for the development of either isolated lung or disseminated disease. See text for discussion. GPL, glycopeptidolipids; LAM, lipoarabinomannans.

production, and increased intracellular survival.[51] Despite the production of a robust proinflammatory response, wild-type serovar 8 and its ssGPL null mutant survived in macrophages. The authors attribute survival of serovar 8 to the production of interleukin 10 (IL-10) by infected macrophages, a response not observed for serovar 2. Clearly, the host response to GPL will depend on the specific NTM serovar responsible for infection.

Lipoglycans

Besides GPL, lipoarabinomannans (LAM) are also recognized virulence factors and are ubiquitous lipids of mycobacteria. However, certain LAM are able to trigger an effective host immune response, to the ultimate detriment of the mycobacteria. LAM consist of 3 structural domains: a carbohydrate backbone and 2 cores (mannan and arabinan). Various caps covering the arabinan classify the 3 heterogenic types of LAM molecules: (1) those with small mannosylated caps are ManLAM (found

in pathogenic *M tuberculosis, M leprae,* and NTM, such as *M avium*), (2) those with phosphatidylinositol caps are PILAM (found in *M fortuitum* and *M smegmatis*), and (3) those without caps are arabinose-capped LAM (AraLAM) (found in *M chelonae*).[52]

The interactions between NTM-derived ManLAM, PILAM, or AraLAM and the host immune response have been partly described. Maeda and colleagues[53] demonstrated that the pattern-recognition receptor Dendritic Cell-Specific Intercellular adhesion molecule-3-Grabbing Non-integrin (DC-SIGN) binds poorly to *M avium* ManLAM containing a single mannose residue, *M fortuitum* PILAM, or uncapped *M chelonae* AraLAM, whereas the 2 to 3 mannose caps of *M tuberculosis* ManLAM are readily recognized by DC-SIGN.[53] PILAM purified from rapidly growing NTM induce the production of proinflammatory cytokines IL-12, TNFα, and IL-8 from differentiated THP-1 human macrophages.[54] Purified AraLAM from *M smegmatis* administered into the lungs of genetically modified mice triggered an acute inflammatory response and neutrophil influx essential to the clearance of *M smegmatis*.[55]

Other mycobacterial lipids (and lipoproteins) of the NTM cell envelope may play a role in enhancing pathogenesis and disease progression. However, until each component is individually purified from the different NTM species and their biological activities systematically scrutinized, the functional role of NTM lipids remains largely unknown.

SUMMARY

In summary, multiple factors are necessary for the pathogenesis of NTM lung disease, including sufficient environmental exposure, host susceptibility factors, and mycobacterial virulence factors. In patients without an obvious host risk factor, the observation that a significant number possess a unique body morphotype and immunophenotype suggests an unidentified host risk factor. The contribution of NTM-derived cell envelope lipids to the pathogenesis of NTM lung disease needs further exploration.

REFERENCES

1. Kim YM, Kim M, Kim SK, et al. Mycobacterial infections in coal workers' pneumoconiosis patients in South Korea. Scand J Infect Dis 2009;41:656–62.

2. Rosenzweig DY. Pulmonary mycobacterial infections due to *Mycobacterium intracellulare-avium* complex. Clinical features and course in 100 consecutive cases. Chest 1979;75:115–9.

3. Sonnenberg P, Murray J, Glynn JR, et al. Risk factors for pulmonary disease due to culture-positive *M. tuberculosis* or non-tuberculous mycobacteria in South African gold miners. Eur Respir J 2000;15:291–6.

4. Chan ED, Kaminska AM, Gill W, et al. Alpha-1-antitrypsin (AAT) anomalies are associated with lung disease due to rapidly growing mycobacteria and AAT inhibits *Mycobacterium abscessus* infection of macrophages. Scand J Infect Dis 2007;39:690–6.

5. Noone PG, Leigh MW, Sannuti A, et al. Primary ciliary dyskinesia: diagnostic and phenotypic features. Am J Respir Crit Care Med 2004;169:459–67.

6. Tomii K, Iwata T, Oida K, et al. A probable case of adult Williams-Campbell syndrome incidentally detected by an episode of atypical mycobacterial infection. Nihon Kyobu Shikkan Gakkai Zasshi 1989;27:518–22.

7. Uji M, Matsushita H, Watanabe T, et al. A case of primary Sjögren's syndrome presenting with middle lobe syndrome complicated by nontuberculous mycobacteriosis. Nihon Kokyuki Gakkai Zasshi 2008;46:55–9.

8. Witty LA, Tapson VF, Piantadosi CA. Isolation of mycobacteria in patients with pulmonary alveolar proteinosis. Medicine 1994;73:103–9.

9. Griffith DE, Girard WM, Wallace RJ. Clinical features of pulmonary disease caused by rapidly growing mycobacteria: an analysis of 154 patients. Am Rev Respir Dis 1993;147:1271–8.

10. Okumura M, Iwai K, Ogata H, et al. Clinical factors on cavitary and nodular bronchiectatic types in pulmonary *Mycobacterium avium* complex disease. Intern Med 2008;47:1465–72.

11. Prince DS, Peterson DD, Steiner RM, et al. Infection with *Mycobacterium avium* complex in patients without predisposing conditions. N Engl J Med 1989;321:863–8.

12. Chan ED, Iseman MD. Slender, older women appear to be more susceptible to nontuberculous mycobacterial lung disease. Gend Med 2010;7:5–18.

13. Iseman MD, Buschman DL, Ackerson LM. Pectus excavatum and scoliosis. Thoracic anomalies associated with pulmonary disease caused by *Mycobacterium avium* complex. Am Rev Respir Dis 1991;144:914–6.

14. Kim RD, Greenberg DE, Ehrmantraut ME, et al. Pulmonary nontuberculous mycobacterial disease: prospective study of a distinct preexisting syndrome. Am J Respir Crit Care Med 2008;178:1066–74.

15. Tasaka S, Hasegawa N, Nishimura T, et al. Elevated serum adiponectin level in patients with *Mycobacterium avium-intracellulare* complex pulmonary disease. Respiration 2010;79:383–7.

16. Lord GM, Matarese G, Howard JK, et al. Leptin modulates the T-cell immune response and reverses starvation-induced immunosuppression. Nature 1998;394:897–901.

17. Ordway D, Henao-Tamayo M, Smith E, et al. Animal model of *Mycobacterium abscessus* lung infection. J Leukoc Biol 2008;83:1502–11.

18. Kartalija M, Ovrutsky AR, Bryan CL, et al. Patients with non-tuberculous mycobacterial lung disease exhibit unique body and immune phenotypes. Am J Respir Crit Care Med 2012;187:197–205.

19. Judge DP, Dietz HC. Marfan's syndrome. Lancet 2005;366:1965–76.

20. Champsi J, Young LS, Bermudez LE. Production of TNF-alpha, IL-6 and TGF-beta, and expression of receptors for TNF-alpha and IL-6, during murine *Mycobacterium avium* infection. Immunology 1995;84:549–54.

21. Denis M, Ghadirian E. Transforming growth factor beta (TGF-b1) plays a detrimental role in the progression of experimental *Mycobacterium avium* infection; in vivo and in vitro evidence. Microb Pathog 1991;11:367–72.

22. Paulson ML, Olivier KN, Holland SM. Pulmonary non-tuberculous mycobacterial infection in congenital contractural arachnodactyly. Int J Tuberc Lung Dis 2012;16:561–3.

23. Tsuyuguchi K, Suzuki K, Matsumoto H, et al. Effect of oestrogen on *Mycobacterium avium* complex pulmonary infection in mice. Clin Exp Immunol 2001;123:428–34.

24. Colombo RE, Hill SC, Claypool RJ, et al. Familial clustering of pulmonary nontuberculous mycobacterial disease. Chest 2010;137:629–34.

25. Fowler CJ, Olivier KN, Leung JM, et al. Abnormal nasal nitric oxide production, ciliary beat frequency, and Toll-like receptor response in pulmonary nontuberculous mycobacterial disease epithelium. Am J Respir Crit Care Med 2013;187:1374–81.

26. Fujita J, Ohtsuki Y, Suemitsu I, et al. Pathological and radiological changes in resected lung specimens in *Mycobacterium avium intracellulare* complex disease. Eur Respir J 1999;13:535–40.

27. Kim TS, Koh WJ, Han J, et al. Hypothesis on the evolution of cavitary lesions in nontuberculous mycobacterial pulmonary infection: thin-section CT and histopathologic correlation. AJR Am J Roentgenol 2005;184:1247–52.

28. Moore EH. Atypical mycobacterial infection in the lung: CT appearance. Radiology 1993;187:777–82.

29. Chan ED, Iseman MD. Bronchiectasis. In: Broaddus EJ, King TE, Lazarus SC, et al, editors. Textbook of respiratory medicine. 6th edition. Elsevier Press; in press.

30. Malcolm KC, Nichols EM, Caceres SM, et al. *Mycobacterium abscessus* induces a limited pattern of neutrophil activation that promotes pathogen survival. PLoS One 2013;8:e57402.

31. McGarvey J, Bermudez LE. Pathogenesis of nontuberculous mycobacteria infections. Clin Chest Med 2002;23:569–83.

32. Rose SJ, Bermudez LE. *Mycobacterium avium* biofilm attenuates mononuclear phagocyte function by triggering hyperstimulation and apoptosis during early infection. Infect Immun 2014;82:405–12.

33. Puzo G. The carbohydrate- and lipid-containing cell wall of mycobacteria, phenolic glycolipids: structure and immunological properties. Crit Rev Microbiol 1990;17:305–27.

34. Pourshafie MR, Sonnenfeld G, Barrow WW. Immunological and ultrastructural disruptions of T lymphocytes following exposure to the glycopeptidolipid isolated from the *Mycobacterium avium* complex. Scand J Immunol 1999;49:405–10.

35. Barrow WW, de Sousa JP, Davis TL, et al. Immunomodulation of human peripheral blood mononuclear cell functions by defined lipid fractions of *Mycobacterium avium*. Infect Immun 1993;61:5286–93.

36. Enomoto K, Oka S, Fujiwara N, et al. Rapid serodiagnosis of *Mycobacterium avium-intracellulare* complex infection by ELISA with cord factor (trehalose 6, 6'-dimycolate), and serotyping using the glycopeptidolipid antigen. Microbiol Immunol 1998;42:689–96.

37. Chatterjee D, Khoo KH. The surface glycopeptidolipids of mycobacteria: structures and biological properties. Cell Mol Life Sci 2001;58:2018–42.

38. Freeman R, Geier H, Weigel KM, et al. Roles for cell wall glycopeptidolipid in surface adherence and planktonic dispersal of *Mycobacterium avium*. Appl Environ Microbiol 2006;72:7554–8.

39. Howard ST, Rhoades E, Recht J, et al. Spontaneous reversion of *Mycobacterium abscessus* from a smooth to a rough morphotype is associated with reduced expression of glycopeptidolipid and reacquisition of an invasive phenotype. Microbiology 2006;152:1581–90.

40. Byrd TF, Lyons CR. Preliminary characterization of a *Mycobacterium abscessus* mutant in human and murine models of infection. Infect Immun 1999;67:4700–7.

41. Rhoades ER, Archambault AS, Greendyke R, et al. *Mycobacterium abscessus* glycopeptidolipids mask underlying cell wall phosphatidyl-myo-inositol mannosides blocking induction of human macrophage TNF-alpha by preventing interaction with TLR2. J Immunol 2009;183:1997–2007.

42. Catherinot E, Roux AL, Macheras E, et al. Acute respiratory failure involving an R variant of *Mycobacterium abscessus*. J Clin Microbiol 2009;47:271–4.

43. Sanguinetti M, Ardito F, Fiscarelli E, et al. Fatal pulmonary infection due to multidrug-resistant *Mycobacterium abscessus* in a patient with cystic fibrosis. J Clin Microbiol 2001;39:816–9.

44. Pawlik A, Garnier G, Orgeur M, et al. Identification and characterization of the genetic changes responsible for the characteristic smooth-to-rough morphotype alterations of clinically persistent *Mycobacterium abscessus*. Mol Microbiol 2013;90:612–29.

45. Pang L, Tian X, Pan W, et al. Structure and function of mycobacterium glycopeptidolipids from comparative genomics perspective. J Cell Biochem 2013;114:1705–13.

46. Sweet L, Schorey JS. Glycopeptidolipids from *Mycobacterium avium* promote macrophage activation in a TLR2- and MyD88-dependent manner. J Leukoc Biol 2006;80:415–23.

47. Barrow WW, Davis TL, Wright EL, et al. Immunomodulatory spectrum of lipids associated with *Mycobacterium avium* serovar 8. Infect Immun 1995;63:126–33.

48. Takegaki Y. Effect of serotype specific glycopeptidolipid (GPL) isolated from *Mycobacterium avium* complex (MAC) on phagocytosis and phagosome-lysosome fusion of human peripheral blood monocytes. Kekkaku 2000;75:9–18.

49. Bhatnagar S, Schorey JS. Exosomes released from infected macrophages contain *Mycobacterium avium* glycopeptidolipids and are proinflammatory. J Biol Chem 2007;282:25779–89.

50. Tereletsky MJ, Barrow WW. Postphagocytic detection of glycopeptidolipids associated with the superficial L1 layer of Mycobacterium intracellulare. Infect Immun 1983;41:1312–21.

51. Cebula BR, Rocco JM, Maslow JN, et al. Mycobacterium avium serovars 2 and 8 infections elicit unique activation of the host macrophage immune responses. Eur J Clin Microbiol Infect Dis 2012;31: 3407–12.

52. Chatterjee D, Khoo KH. Mycobacterial lipoarabinomannan: an extraordinary lipoheteroglycan with profound physiological effects. Glycobiology 1998;8: 113–20.

53. Maeda N, Nigou J, Herrmann JL, et al. The cell surface receptor DC-SIGN discriminates between Mycobacterium species through selective recognition of the mannose caps on lipoarabinomannan. J Biol Chem 2003;278:5513–6.

54. Vignal C, Guerardel Y, Kremer L, et al. Lipomannans, but not lipoarabinomannans, purified from Mycobacterium chelonae and Mycobacterium kansasii induce TNF-alpha and IL-8 secretion by a CD14-toll-like receptor 2-dependent mechanism. J Immunol 2003;171:2014–23.

55. Wieland CW, Knapp S, Florquin S, et al. Non-mannose-capped lipoarabinomannan induces lung inflammation via toll-like receptor 2. Am J Respir Crit Care Med 2004;170:1367–74.

56. Winthrop KL, Baxter R, Liu L, et al. Mycobacterial diseases and antitumour necrosis factor therapy in USA. Ann Rheum Dis 2013;72:37–42.

57. Doucette K, Fishman JA. Nontuberculous mycobacterial infection in hematopoietic stem cell and solid organ transplant recipients. Clin Infect Dis 2004; 38:1428–39.

58. French AL, Benator DA, Gordin FM. Nontuberculous mycobacterial infections. Med Clin North Am 1997; 81:361–79.

59. Dorman SE, Picard C, Lammas D, et al. Clinical features of dominant and recessive interferon gamma receptor 1 deficiencies. Lancet 2004;364:2113–21.

60. Döffinger R, Jouanguy E, Dupuis S, et al. Partial interferon-gamma receptor signaling chain deficiency in a patient with bacille Calmette-Guérin and Mycobacterium abscessus infection. J Infect Dis 2000;181:379–84.

61. Dupuis S, Dargemont C, Fieschi C, et al. Impairment of mycobacterial but not viral immunity by a germline human STAT1 mutation. Science 2001;293:300–3.

62. Prando C, Samarina A, Bustamante J, et al. Inherited IL-12p40 deficiency: genetic, immunologic, and clinical features of 49 patients from 30 kindreds. Medicine (Baltimore) 2013;92:109–22.

63. Haverkamp MH, van de Vosse E, van Dissel JT. Non-tuberculous mycobacterial infections in children with inborn errors of the immune system. J Infect 2014; 68:S134–50.

64. Minegishi Y, Saito M, Morio T, et al. Human tyrosine kinase 2 deficiency reveals its requisite roles in multiple cytokine signals involved in innate and acquired immunity. Immunity 2006;25:745–55.

65. Filipe-Santos O, Bustamante J, Haverkamp MH, et al. X-linked susceptibility to mycobacteria is caused by mutations in NEMO impairing CD40-dependent IL-12 production. J Exp Med 2006;203: 1745–59.

66. Chi CY, Chu CC, Liu JP, et al. Anti-IFN-γ autoantibodies in adults with disseminated nontuberculous mycobacterial infections are associated with HLA-DRB1*16:02 and HLA-DQB1*05:02 and the reactivation of latent varicella-zoster virus infection. Blood 2013;121:1357–66.

67. Hsu AP, Johnson KD, Falcone EL, et al. GATA2 haploinsufficiency caused by mutations in a conserved intronic element leads to MonoMAC syndrome. Blood 2013;121:3830–7.

68. Bustamante J, Arias AA, Vogt G, et al. Germline CYBB mutations that selectively affect macrophages in kindreds with X-linked predisposition to tuberculous mycobacterial disease. Nat Immunol 2011;12: 213–21.

69. Bogunovic D, Byun M, Durfee LA, et al. Mycobacterial disease and impaired IFN-γ immunity in humans with inherited ISG15 deficiency. Science 2012;337: 1684–8.

70. Hambleton S, Salem S, Bustamante J, et al. IRF8 mutations and human dendritic-cell immunodeficiency. N Engl J Med 2011;365:127–38.

Epidemiology of Human Pulmonary Infection with Nontuberculous Mycobacteria
A Review

D. Rebecca Prevots, PhD, MPH[a],*,
Theodore K. Marras, MD, MSc[b]

KEYWORDS

- Epidemiology • Nontuberculous mycobacteria • Pulmonary disease • Global

KEY POINTS

- Population-based data from North America, Europe, and Australia show that the prevalence of non-tuberculous mycobacteria (NTM)-related pulmonary disease (NTM PD) continues to increase, and that prevalence is lower in Europe than in North America and Australia.
- Large tertiary care facility–based studies in East Asia (Japan, South Korea, Taiwan) also suggest high and increasing prevalence of NTM PD.
- In selected African countries, NTM were identified in 4.2% to 15% of suspected tuberculosis (TB) cases and in 18% to 20% of persons with "chronic" suspected multidrug-resistant TB.
- Improved surveillance for NTM is needed, including population-based surveillance and sentinel studies.
- Host and environmental factors interact in disease risk; host factors include neoplasms, preexisting lung disease, and more recently identified factors such as thoracic skeletal abnormalities, rheumatoid arthritis, and immunomodulatory drugs. Environmental risk factors for disease clustering include high vapor pressure such as is found in warm, humid environments.

INTRODUCTION

This article reviews approaches to studying the epidemiology of nontuberculous mycobacteria (NTM)-related pulmonary disease (NTM PD), and updates in the field since the last review published in 2002.[1]

Methodologic Challenges

Studying the epidemiology of NTM PD presents several methodologic challenges that affect the measures obtained. First, with a few exceptions,[2]

in most countries NTM PD is not a reportable condition, such that describing the burden, trends, and associated risk factors for this condition depend on special studies, surveys, and sentinel surveillance efforts described later in this article. Second, isolation from an uncontaminated clinical specimen is insufficient to document disease, because respiratory secretions from patients with underlying lung disease may be colonized with these organisms without overt untoward manifestations For this reason, clinical information is required in concert with microbiological data to

Disclosures: None.
[a] Epidemiology Unit, Laboratory of Clinical Infectious Diseases, Division of Intramural Research, National Institute of Allergy and Infectious Diseases, National Institutes of Health, 9000 Rockville Pike, Building 15B-1, 8 West Drive, MSC 2665, Bethesda, MD 20892, USA; [b] Division of Respirology, Department of Medicine, University of Toronto and Toronto Western Hospital, 399 Bathurst Street, 7E-452, Toronto, ON M5T 2S8, Canada
* Corresponding author.
E-mail address: rprevots@niaid.nih.gov

Clin Chest Med 36 (2015) 13–34
http://dx.doi.org/10.1016/j.ccm.2014.10.002
0272-5231/15/$ – see front matter Published by Elsevier Inc.

be certain whether disease is present in an individual, although reliance on solely microbiological information has recently been shown to provide a reasonable approximation.[3–5] The diagnosis comprises 3 components to include microbiological, radiographic, and clinical criteria.[6] These criteria require that a patient with symptoms seeks health care, that the health care provider suspects a diagnosis, that appropriate samples are obtained (sputum or lung biopsy), and that radiographic imaging is performed. Finally, the disease is often indolent (slowly progressive) and chronic, and patients may not be routinely evaluated with appropriate samples throughout their disease course. Often patients may have difficulty producing sputum samples, which limits the ability to obtain appropriate samples. In one study of NTM, 40% to 70% of patients were cultured in only a single year during a study period spanning from 5 to beyond 10 years.[3]

Measures of Disease Burden

For a chronic disease such as NTM PD, prevalence is the best measure of disease burden in a population. Incidence is a measure of the frequency of new infections and is the best measure for identifying risk factors for disease. Defining incidence, that is, the frequency of new cases occurring in a defined population over a specified time period, requires definition of a time period when patients were disease-free. Because the disease is often indolent and samples for microbiological analysis may not be taken, this disease-free risk window may not be clear.

Prevalence is a measure of the frequency of all cases existent in a defined population, newly or previously diagnosed. Two measures of prevalence have been used to define the NTM PD burden in a population: average annual prevalence and period prevalence.[3,4,7,8] The average annual prevalence is defined by averaging the annual number of cases over a defined period and dividing by the average annual population over that time period. The period prevalence is defined as the total number of cases existent over a defined period divided by the population in that time period. For a longer time period, for example over 5 to 10 years, the period prevalence estimates will always be greater than an average annual population estimate because for the former, cases are summed over multiple years so that cases that are identified only once during a period of interest whereas for annual prevalence, the same case occurring over multiple years would be counted only in years in which multiple isolates are obtained, despite ongoing chronic disease.

Although mortality data are suboptimal given the uncertain validity of death certificate coding for NTM PD as a cause of death, such data have been used in 2 instances to provide a national picture of the epidemiology of NTM. In the United States, mortality patterns mirrored prevalence data with respect to time, place, and person.[9] In Japan, mortality data were useful for providing insight into patterns by age, sex, and region, and for estimating prevalence.[10]

Risk Factors: Approaches

To more fully understand the population patterns and trends for NTM PD, both host and environmental risk factors must be considered, as both contribute to disease patterns. Because these organisms are widespread in soil and water in most countries and yet disease is rare, host susceptibility likely plays a key role. The role of inherited genetic factors can be studied by both traditional and modern genetic methods. Traditional methods include pedigree analysis to indicate clustering of NTM PD and related traits within families.[11,12] Future studies can include approaches such as whole-exome sequencing or candidate gene approaches to identify variants associated with disease or severe disease, similar to the work that has been done for cystic fibrosis (CF) to identify genetic modifiers of disease.[13] For studies involving genetic sequencing, as with any control group, the comparison population should be as similar as possible to the case group except with respect to the factor under study. Characterization of human leukocyte antigen types has also been used to identify genetic variants associated with NTM disease.[14,15]

An area of great concern has been the role of specific environmental exposures to soil and water, and particularly to water aerosols from showers and baths.[16] One approach to studying this has been to design case-control studies with detailed ascertainment of these exposures. However, the measurement of individual behaviors is limited by recall bias and the unknown incubation period (time between exposure and disease onset). In addition, these studies are limited to some degree by the lack of knowledge regarding infectious dose for NTM PD, which would help guide the detail needed for exposure ascertainment. An alternative and more recent approach has been to study these factors using spatial analysis, which allows detection of disease clusters and analysis of the association of these clusters with atmospheric and other environmental conditions.[17,18] Because NTM are environmental organisms, an analytical approach that seeks to relate population patterns to environmental conditions may be a better approach, as these factors act beyond the individual (ie, influencing mycobacteria grown in and near bodies of water) in a truly ecologic fashion.

Host and Environmental Risk Factors: Findings

Host and environmental risk factors identified to date are summarized in **Table 1**. Case-control

Table 1
Risk factors for NTM infection and disease

Risk Factor	Relative Risk, Odds Ratio, or Relative Prevalence	Disease or Infection
Environmental: individual exposures		
Soil exposure	5.9[21]	Disease
Indoor swimming pool use (in the past 4 mo)	5.9 (1.3, 26.1)[20]	Infection
Swimming pool use at least once per month (indoor or outdoor, over the past 5 y)	0.15 (0.04–0.67)[19]	Disease
Host factors		
Lung cancer (neoplasms of larynx, trachea, and bronchus)	3.4[7]	Disease
COPD	2–10[7,19,27]	Disease
Bronchiectasis	44–187.5[7,23]	Disease (coding)[7] Disease (validated microbiological surrogate)[23]
Thoracic skeletal abnormalities	5.4[19]	Disease
Low body weight	9.09[a,19]	Disease
Rheumatoid arthritis	1.5,[7] 1.9[b,26]	Disease
Immunomodulatory drugs/anti-TNF agents	OR = infinity[19] Anti-TNF agents 2.2[78] Others 1.6–2.9[78]	Disease
Steroid use	8[19] 1.6[78]	Disease
Gastroesophageal reflux disease	5.3[c,27] 1.5[a,26]	Disease
Environmental: climatic and population factors		
Proportion of area as surface water	4.6[17]	Disease
Mean daily potential evapotranspiration	4.0[17]	Disease
Copper soil levels, per 1 ppm increase	1.2 (1.0, 1.2)[17]	Disease
Sodium soil levels, per 0.1 ppm increase	1.9 (1.2, 2.9)[17]	Disease
Manganese soil levels, per 100 ppm increase	0.7 (0.4, 1.0)[17]	Disease
Increased average topsoil depth	0.87 (*Mycobacterium intracellulare*)[18]	Disease
Soil bulk density	1.8 (*Mycobacterium kansasii*)[18]	Disease

Abbreviations: COPD, chronic obstructive pulmonary disease; OR, odds ratio; TNF, tumor necrosis factor.
[a] Estimated from data in article.
[b] Hazard ratio, fully adjusted for age, sex, income, rurality, and comorbidities for NTM (human immunodeficiency virus, COPD, asthma, and gastrointestinal reflux disease).
[c] Comparison of cases and non-cases among anti-TNF users.

studies that have attempted to identify environmental and host factors associated with disease have had somewhat inconsistent results, likely attributable to both methodologic and population differences. One study in the United States, which measured exposure to both soil and water aerosol in addition to host factors, found several host factors with significant associations with disease, whereas few to no environmental exposures were identified as risk factors.[19] In this study the only important protective factors identified were any swimming pool use (indoor or outdoor) and washing dishes by hand. However, these effects were considered to be likely due to a bias whereby healthier patients are more likely to engage in these activities.[19] In another case-control study of the risk of environmental exposures for NTM among persons with CF, indoor swimming pool use at least monthly was significantly associated with NTM infection (see **Table 1**).[20] One study in Japan found that exposure to soil more than twice weekly was significantly associated with disease.[21]

Medical host factors are also detailed in **Table 1**. When measures of association are available these are presented, the focus being on comparisons with non-NTM (or tuberculosis [TB]) infected populations. Historically, NTM was associated with neoplasms and structural lung diseases such as chronic obstructive pulmonary disease (COPD),[1] and these underlying diseases remain important predisposing factors for NTM (see **Table 1**). The population affected by COPD has tended to be predominantly male, which reflects to a large degree the patterns of smoking in the population. In countries where smoking remains prevalent, COPD remains an important predisposing risk factor, and detailed later in this article in the regional sections. Persons with CF are disproportionately affected by NTM, with a national prevalence estimated at 13%,[22] and this topic is covered in an article elsewhere in this issue by Drs Martiniano and Nick. In a nationally representative sample of older adults in the United States, bronchiectasis was also strongly associated with NTM PD, although this condition was more prevalent among women with NTM PD than in men with NTM PD.[7] Bronchiectasis was also found to be strongly associated with NTM lung disease in a nationwide study in Denmark, with an odds ratio of 187.5.[23]

In recent decades, coincident with a major increase in NTM, a predominance of women without known risk factors has been observed.[24] In this population with "idiopathic" NTM PD, women with a tall, thin morphotype predominate[25]; recently identified risk factors include thoracic

skeletal abnormalities and low body mass index.[19] Use of immunomodulatory drugs or steroids are also associated with NTM PD,[19] as is rheumatoid arthritis per se, with risk increasing further in the presence of more potent immunosuppressive therapy (see **Table 1**).[26,27] No consistent association with diabetes and NTM PD has been found.[7,19,27]

Although individual factors predispose for disease, an interaction with environmental conditions clearly exists.[28] In the United States, both *Mycobacterium intracellulare* skin-test sensitization[29] and NTM PD are more prevalent in the warmer, more humid areas of the Southeast and Southwest. In Japan, NTM PD mortality, a surrogate measure of disease prevalence and distribution, has a higher prevalence in the warmer and more humid coastal areas and in an area with a large lake. Recent studies have used geospatial approaches to identify climatic factors that influence the population risk of NTM PD. Two studies in the United States have identified atmospheric factors predictive of disease prevalence or disease clustering in a geographic area (see **Table 1**). Prevots and colleagues[20,28] found that evapotranspiration (the potential of the atmosphere to absorb water) and the proportion of the area as surface water were predictive of disease clustering in an area, and both studies found that vapor pressure (a measure of the water in the atmosphere at a given temperature) was predictive of disease prevalence among CF patients. These population findings are consistent with an earlier environmental microbiology study which found that warmer temperature, low pH, low dissolved oxygen, high soluble zinc, high humic acid, and high fulvic acid are related to the environmental prevalence of NTM.[30] In Queensland, Australia, in one of the few epidemiologic studies to evaluate environmental factors by species, increased average topsoil depth was protective against *M intracellulare*, whereas increased soil bulk density was positively associated with *Mycobacterium kansasii* disease (see **Table 1**).[18]

Prevalence and Incidence

In areas where NTM is reportable, such as the province of Queensland, Australia,[2] data based on isolates linked to clinical information provide a representative pattern of disease by time, place, and person. Sentinel surveillance comprises a single site or sample of sites that voluntarily report data on isolates, with a standard set of clinical information collected for patients. If the surveillance network is nationally representative, this system can provide good prevalence estimates.

One example is the mycobacterial study group in France, which reported data on NTM isolates and associated clinical information during a 3-year period.[31]

Several other types of prevalence studies have been published, which include those limited to microbiological isolation, those with microbiological and limited clinical information, and those with complete clinical information (fully defined). For example, the NTM-Network of the European Trials Group (NET) compiles species information from isolates throughout participating laboratories in Europe and elsewhere. A strength of this collaboration is the number of isolates and participating countries, and the data provide a snapshot of the species distribution across regions and countries.[33] This measure would likely overestimate disease prevalence, as not all persons with 1 or more isolates will meet American Thoracic Society (ATS) disease criteria. Similarly, regional laboratories with complete capture of a defined geographic region and population, such as provincial laboratories in Canada,[8] can also provide a representative picture of isolates.

When surveillance or regionally representative data are not available, other approaches can provide a representative picture. An ideal study type is one that has electronic laboratory data linked to clinical data and other diagnostic information in a defined population, such as that available for integrated health care delivery systems in the United States,[3] or integrated health care systems in other countries. When laboratory data are not available, International Diagnostic Classification of Diseases, 9th revision (ICD-9) codes provide a surrogate measure of diagnosis and are useful for estimating the prevalence of this rare condition from large administrative data sets such as Medicare.[7] Estimates for the sensitivity of ICD-9 codes vary from 27% to 50%.[3,27,32] Although these codes underestimate the true prevalence of NTM, this bias is not likely to be systematic; therefore, these codes provide an important tool for estimating prevalence by demographic features and comorbid conditions. Within these various approaches to estimating prevalence, study populations may be regionally representative,[33] nationally representative,[7] or representative of an area or state within a country.[3,34]

EPIDEMIOLOGY OF NONTUBERCULOUS MYCOBACTERIA ISOLATION AND DISEASE BY GLOBAL REGION

In this review of epidemiologic data of pulmonary NTM, the aim is to include the highest-quality data published since 2000. Ideal studies comprise population-based investigations including both clinical and microbiological data, and encompassing an adequate temporal period to best capture the burden of infection in the population. Reviews of the best available studies by global region are presented.

North America

The study of pulmonary NTM epidemiology in North America has advanced substantially in recent years. Numerous studies that are either population based or from epidemiologically relevant population subgroups have been published, and several studies have provided estimates of period prevalence in addition to annual prevalence. Studies focusing exclusively on hospitalized patients, or in which case-identification criteria are deemed inadequate, are excluded. Included are studies presenting data from a single institution for the assessment of relative species frequency and for information regarding population patterns including age, sex, and preexisting lung disease. **Table 2** presents results regarding the frequency of NTM PD while **Table 3** presents data regarding relative frequency of different species among populations with NTM PD.

Comprehensive population-based studies in Ontario, Canada have demonstrated annual rates of isolation prevalence of 14.1 to 22.2 per 100,000 population.[8,35,36] Because these studies were limited by a lack of clinical information, a surrogate microbiological definition of disease was used ($\geq$2 positive sputum samples or $\geq$1 positive bronchoscopic or biopsy sample). In one of these studies, annual disease prevalence was estimated at 9.8/100,000 in 2010 while period prevalence of disease was estimated at 41.3/100,000 over the 5-year period 2006 to 2010.[8] All of these studies excluded *Mycobacterium gordonae*. In Ontario, *Mycobacterium avium* complex (MAC) was most commonly isolated and identified as a cause of disease, followed by *Mycobacterium xenopi* and the rapidly growing mycobacteria (RGM) (see **Table 2**). These data offer accurate estimates of isolation prevalence in a population of approximately 13 million people, but estimates of disease were limited by the lack of clinical information.

Following implementation of statewide NTM isolation reporting for 2005 to 2006, and using standardized protocols for NTM case investigation, investigators in Oregon, USA described NTM epidemiology in a comprehensive statewide microbiologically based study, with complete clinical record reviews among a subset of subjects in the Portland area.[4,34] Excluding *M gordonae*, annualized isolation prevalence of pulmonary

Table 2
Studies of rates of pulmonary NTM isolation and disease by region

Location (Dates)	Disease Definition	Annual Rates[a] (Species Frequency)		Period Prevalence of Disease	
		Isolation	Disease	Period Duration (y)	Prevalence
North America					
Oregon, USA (2005–2006)[34,b]	Microbiological	12.7	5.6	2	11.1
Portland, Oregon, USA (2005–2006)[4,b]	Microbiological and clinical	NR	NR	2	8.6 (general population)[c] 20.4 (age ≥50 y)[c] MAC 87.5% Mycobacterium abscessus/ chelonae 6%
Beneficiaries of 4 integrated health care delivery systems in California, Colorado, Pennsylvania, and Washington, USA (2004–2006)[3,b]	Microbiological results with ICD-9 coding with subset clinical review for validation	11.8 (all sites combined)	5.5 (all sites combined)	3	<60 y ~4 60–69 y ~40 70–79 y ~100 ≥80 y ~220
Ontario, Canada (1997–2007)[36,b]	NA	19.2	NR	NA	NR
USA (nationwide) Medicare beneficiaries (≥65 y of age) (1997–2007)[7]	ICD-9 coding	NA	~47	≤11	≥65 y = 112
Ontario, Canada (1998–2010)[8,b]	Microbiological	22.2	9.8	5	41.3 (2006–2010)

Location (Dates)	Disease Definition	Annual Rates (Species Frequency)		Period Prevalence of Disease[e]	
		Isolation[d]	Disease[d]	Period Duration (y)	Prevalence[d]
Central and South America					
Baixada Santista region, São Paulo, Brazil (2000–2005)[39]	Microbiological	Total 1.31 HIV negative 0.77 HIV positive 0.55	Total 0.25	6	1.5
São Jose do Rio Preto, Brazil (1996–2005)[40]	Microbiological	5.3	1.0	10	10

Location (Dates)	Disease Definition	Annual Rates (Species Frequency)		Period Prevalence of Disease[e]	
		Isolation	Disease	Period Duration (y)	Prevalence
Europe					
Southwest Ireland (1987–2000)[44]	Microbiological and clinical	1.9	0.2	NA	NR
Borders region, Scotland (1992–2010)[50]	Microbiological; subset clinical	NR	0.86 (1992–2004) 3.1 (2005–2010)	NR	NR
Leeds, UK (1995–1999)[46]	Microbiological and clinical	2.9	1.7	5	8.5
Denmark, nationwide (1997–2008)[5]	Microbiological; subset clinical	2.5	1.1	12	5–8
Nijmegen-Arnhem region, Netherlands (1999–2005)[48]	Microbiological and clinical	6.3	1.4	7	9.8
France, multisite (2000–2002)[33,f]	Microbiological and clinical	MAC 0.4	MAC 0.2	3	0.6
Crete, Greece (2000–2009)[49]	Microbiological; subset clinical	NR	0.6	NA	NR
France, multisite (2001–2003)[45,f]	Microbiological and clinical	NR	0.73	3	2.2
Central Greece (2004–2006)[47]	Microbiological and clinical	7.0	0.7	3	2.1
Croatia, nationwide (2006–2010)[51]	Microbiological	5.3	0.75	3	2.1

Location (Dates)	Disease Definition	Annual Rates[a] (Species Frequency)		Period Prevalence of Disease[e]	
		Isolation	Disease	Period Duration	Prevalence
Australia					
Australia, national (2000)[76]	Microbiological and clinical	5.9	0.56	NA	NR
Queensland, Australia, statewide (1999–2005)[2]	Microbiological and clinical	NR	3.2	NA	NR
New Zealand, national (2004)[77]	Microbiological and clinical	3.77	0.56	NA	NR

Abbreviations: HIV, human immunodeficiency virus; ICD-9, International Diagnostic Classification of Diseases, 9th revision; MAC, *Mycobacterium avium* complex; NA, not available; NR, not reported.

[a] Rates expressed as annual rates per 100,000 population, averaged over study period unless otherwise specified.
[b] Studies that excluded *Mycobacterium gordonae*.
[c] Prevalence figures represent underestimates: 30% of records unavailable to determine disease status.
[d] Based on assumption of population-based study.
[e] Estimated from data in reports.
[f] Sentinel-site methodology used to extrapolate multisite prevalence estimates over entire nation.

Table 3
NTM lung disease by species and region

Location (Dates)	N		Most Common Species			
North America						
New York City, USA single institution (2000–2004)[79]	81	MAC (80%)	Mycobacterium abscessus/chelonae (13%)	Mycobacterium fortuitum (8%)	Mycobacterium xenopi (6%)	Mycobacterium kansasii (5%)
Oregon, USA, statewide population-based (2005–2006)[34]	407	MAC (85%)	M abscessus/chelonae (4%)	Mycobacterium xenopi (1%)	M fortuitum (<1%)	Mycobacterium goodi (<1%)
Toronto, Canada, single institution (2002–2003)[37]	255	MAC (69%)	M xenopi (21%)	RGM (7%)		
Four integrated health care delivery systems, USA, in California, Colorado, Pennsylvania, and Washington (1994–2006)[3]	1865	MAC (80%)	M abscessus/chelonae (12%)	M fortuitum (6%)	M kansasii (6%)	Mycobacterium simiae (3%)
Charlottesville, Virginia, USA, single institution (2001–2009)[38]	83	MAC (69%)	M kansasii (5%)	M xenopi (5%)	M abscessus (4%)	M fortuitum (4%)
Ontario, Canada (2010)[8]	1294	MAC (64%)	M xenopi (23%)	M abscessus (3%)	M fortuitum (3%)	
Central and South America						
Baixada Santista region, São Paulo, Brazil (2000–2005)[39]	125	M kansasii (20.8%)	MAC (20%)	M fortuitum (16%)		
São Jose do Rio Preto, Brazil (1996–2005)[40]	184	MAC (62.9%)	M fortuitum (11.4%)	M gordonae (8.5%)	M chelonae (5.7%)	M kansasii M abscessus (each 2.9%)

	N					
Buenos Aires Province, Argentina (2004–2010)[41]	54	MAC (48%) Mycobacterium avium (20.4%) Mycobacterium intracellulare (27.8%)	M kansasii (13%)	Mycobacterium gordonae (13%)	M fortuitum (3.7%)	Mycobacterium scrofulaceum (3.7%)
Rio de Janeiro, Brazil (1993–2011)[42]	127	MAC (35.4%)	M kansasii (33.1%)	M abscessus (18.9%)	M fortuitum (8.7%)	
Para State, Brazil (2010–2011)[43]	29	Mycobacterium massiliense (44.8%)	MAC (20.7%) M avium (10.3%) M intracellulare (10.3%)	M abscessus (6.9%)	Mycobacterium bolletii, Mycobacterium celatum, M fortuitum, M kansasii, Mycobacterium mariokaense (each 3.4%)	
Europe						
Southwest Ireland (1987–2000)[44]	17	MAC (82%)	M malmoense (12%)	M abscessus (6%)		
France, multisite (2001–2003)[45]	263	MAC (48%)	M xenopi (25%)	M kansasii (13%)	M abscessus (9%)	
Leeds, UK (1995–1999)[46]	49	MAC (45%)	M malmoense (37%)	M xenopi (6%)	M kansasii (6%)	
Nijmegen-Arnhem region, Netherlands (1999–2005)[48]	53	MAC (49%) M avium (45%) M intracellulare (3.8%)	M kansasii (23%)	Mycobacterium szulgai (7.5%)	M xenopi (5.6%)	
Denmark, nationwide (1997–2008)[5]	335	MAC (57%)	M malmoense (8.1%)	M xenopi (7.8%)	M abscessus (6.9%)	M gordonae (5.4%)
Central Greece (2004–2006)[47]	16	M fortuitum (62.5%)	MAC (25%)	M malmoense (12.5%)		
Lisbon, Portugal (2008–2009)[80]	58	MAC (22.4%) M avium (6.9%) M intracellulare (15.5%)	M fortuitum (13.8%)	M gordonae (12.1%)	M kansasii (10.3%)	M chelonae (8.6%)
Naples, Italy (2006–2009)[81]	16	M intracellulare (43.8%)	M kansasii (31.3%)	M xenopi (12.5%)	M fortuitum (6.3%)	

(continued on next page)

Table 3
(continued)

Location (Dates)	N	Most Common Species		
Crete, Greece (2000–2009)[49]	38	MAC (40%)	M kansasii (26%)	M abscessus (8%)	M fortuitum, M chelonae, M gordonae (each 5%)
London, England, single institution (2000–2007, slowly growing NTM)[82]	57	M kansasii (70%)	MAC (40%)	M malmoense (9%)	M xenopi (7%)
Borders region, Scotland (1992–2010)[50]	32	MAC (43.8%)	M malmoense (12.5%)	M chelonae (9.4%)	M gordonae (9.4%)	Mycobacterium nonchromogenicum, Mycobacterium terrae, M xenopi (each 6.3%)
Croatia, nationwide (2006–2010)[51]	167	M xenopi (28.1%)	M gordonae (20.4%)	MAC (19.8%) M avium (14.4%) M intracellulare (5.4%)	M fortuitum (11.4%)
Middle East and South Asia				
Turkey, single institution (2004–2009)[60]	31	MAC (42%) M intracellulare (32%) M avium (10%)	M abscessus (16%)	M kansasii (16%)	
Israel, single institution (2004–2010)[61]	45	M xenopi (29%)	M kansasii (20%)	MAC (18%)	M fortuitum (9%)
Saudi Arabia, sampling of several institutions (2009–2010)[62]	49	M abscessus (30.6%)	M fortuitum (28.6%)	MAC (16.3%) M intracellulare 10.2%) M avium (6.1%)	M kansasii (8.2%)
Oman, sample of NTM lung disease cases from central laboratory (2006–2007)[63]	7	MAC (71.4%) M intracellulare (28.6%) Mycobacterium chimaera (28.6%)	Mycobacterium colombiense (14.3%)	Mycobacterium simiae (14.3%)	

Location (years)	N				
India, single institution (2005–2008)[64]	67	MAC (34%) M intracellulare (22%) M avium (4.5%)	M abscessus (22%)	M simiae (22%)	M fortuitum (12%)
East Asia					
Seoul, South Korea, single institution (2002–2003)[65]	195	MAC (48%) M intracellulare (29%) M avium (19%)	M abscessus (33%)	M fortuitum (11%)	M kansasii (4%)
Seoul, South Korea, single institution (2002–2008)[83]	651	MAC (62.9%)	M abscessus (26.7%)		
Seoul, South Korea, single institution (2006–2010)[84]	345	MAC (76.2%) M avium (40.9%) M intracellulare (35.4%)	M abscessus (18.2%)	M fortuitum (2.3%)	M kansasii (2.0%)
Kaohsiung City, Southern Taiwan, single institution (2004–2005)[71]	67	M abscessus (44.8%)	M fortuitum (23.9%)	MAC (14.9%)	M kansasii (13.4%)
Taipei City, Northern Taiwan, single institution (2007–2009)[73a]	252	MAC (39.7%)	M chelonae-abscessus (30.2%)	M kansasii (11.1%)	M fortuitum (9.5%)
Australia					
Australia, national (2000)[76]	107	MAC (67.3%)	M kansasii (19.6%)	M abscessus (6.5%)	
Queensland, Australia, statewide (1999–2005)[2]	130	MAC (73.8%) M intracellulare (60%) M avium (13.8%)	M kansasii (7.7%)	M abscessus (5.4%)	
New Zealand, national (2004)[77]	47	MAC (83%)	M abscessus (9%)		

Abbreviations: MAC, *Mycobacterium avium* complex; RGM, rapidly growing nontuberculous mycobacterial species.
[a] Included only patients whose radiographic disease pattern could be classified as cavitary, bronochiectatic, or consolidative.

NTM was 12.7/100,000[34] and the 2-year period prevalence of disease, defined by full microbiological and clinical criteria, was estimated at 8.6/100,000.[4] Records were available for review in approximately 70% of subjects in the Portland area, so disease rates were underestimated. The Oregon data offer robust population-based estimates of isolation prevalence in 3.7 million people but, because of the incomplete availability of clinical records, substantially underestimated disease prevalence.

The epidemiology of NTM has been studied in several closed system managed care organizations in the United States. A multicenter study was performed in 4 integrated health care delivery systems, including 4.1 million beneficiaries in California, Colorado, Pennsylvania, and Washington.[3] The investigators extracted microbiological and ICD-9 coded records data, and validated a subset of patients for radiographic evidence of disease. The annual site-specific prevalence of NTM PD (excluding M gordonae) was found to be 1.4 to 6.6 per 100,000. Strengths of these data rest on the diversity of the studied geographic regions and the validation of cases.

A nationwide United States study of Medicare beneficiaries (≥65 years of age) from 1997 through 2007[7] provides valuable insight regarding disease frequency in older adults, who comprise most NTM patients. The investigators used ICD-9 coding to identify cases of NTM disease and observed an annual prevalence of approximately 47/100,000 in 2007. Intriguing geographic heterogeneity was

identified. Regional period prevalence was highest in the West (149/100,000), driven largely by California (191/100,000) and Hawaii (396/100,000), and second highest in the Southeast (131/100,000). In this older adult population, an average annual increase of NTM disease of 8.5% was observed from 1997 to 2007 (**Fig. 1**).[7] In managed care organizations in the United States, increases of nearly 3% per year were observed from 1994 to 2006.[3] In Ontario, Canada, the average increase in annual disease prevalence was 6.3% per year from 1998 to 2010[8] (**Fig. 2**) while the 5-year period prevalence increased from 29.3/100,000 (1998–2002) to 41.3/100,000 (2006–2010).[8]

Information from studies presenting data on the proportion of NTM PD caused by different species is presented in **Table 3**. In all studies, MAC was the most common species complex (64%–85% of cases), followed in most studies by *Mycobacterium abscessus/chelonae* (3%–13%), *M xenopi* (1%–23%), *Mycobacterium fortuitum* (<1%–8%), and *M kansasii* (<1%–6%). Recently, data from various North American centers were compiled as part of a global NTM collaboration.[33]

In North America, most patients tended to be women (range 55%–66%), and were more likely to be older adults (mean age 68.2 years, range 59–70 years) (**Table 4**). Most recent North American studies did not report on whether patients had preexisting lung disease, but the frequency of COPD was described in 4 studies[3,4,37,38] wherein 28% to 66% of patients had COPD (see **Table 4**). With respect to prevalence by racial/

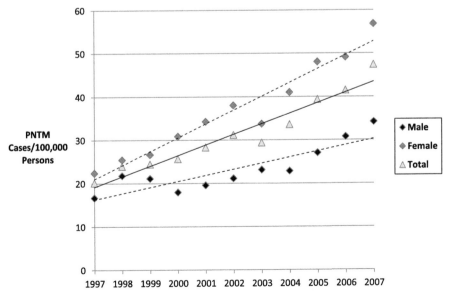

Fig. 1. Annual prevalence of pulmonary nontuberculous mycobacterial infection (PNTM) cases among a sample of US Medicare Part B enrollees by sex, 1997 to 2007.

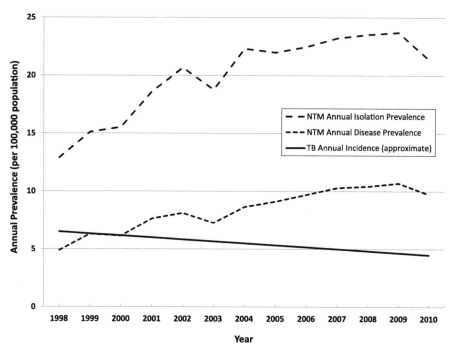

Fig. 2. Prevalence of nontuberculous mycobacteria (NTM) isolation and disease, and incidence of tuberculosis (TB), Canada, 1998 to 2010.

ethnic groups, of interest is the finding that in the United States, among persons aged 65 years and older, persons classified as "Asian" had relative prevalence rates approximately 2-fold higher than persons categorized as "white."

In summary, data from recent North American studies generally suggest annual rates of NTM isolation of 6 to 22 per 100,000, and annual rates of disease of 5 to 10 per 100,000. Period prevalence estimates, undoubtedly a superior measure of the burden of disease, varied widely based on the period duration and age group studied. Period prevalence in studies including all ages ranged from 9 to 41 per 100,000, and was far higher when focusing on older subpopulations. Most studies demonstrated temporal increases in the frequency of NTM PD over a 3- to 11-year period. Limitations included heterogeneous case ascertainment and disease definitions, and incomplete age-group or geographic coverage. In the United States, nationally representative estimates of the population younger than 65 years are not available. In Canada, large geographic areas outside the province of Ontario have not been systematically studied, and there has been limited assessment utilizing clinical record review within Ontario. NTM PD in North America is very strongly associated with increasing age (especially common in the elderly) and COPD, and is reported more commonly in females. The prevalence of

NTM PD varies with both the presence of COPD and gender, whereby men seem to more commonly have secondary NTM, with predisposing COPD, whereas women most commonly appear to have idiopathic NTM.[37]

Central and South America

Several recent studies, generally from single institutions, have added to the understanding of the epidemiology of NTM PD in Central and South America. The limitation common to all of these studies is the lack of a reliable denominator in a defined population, making estimates regarding NTM frequency uncertain. In addition, data regarding species distribution may also be affected by referral bias to the institutions from which data were reported. The latter may be relevant if NTM species varies according to clinical features, such as COPD, or if clinicians' referral may depend on the species isolated and the perception of its pathogenicity. **Table 2** presents results regarding NTM frequency while **Table 3** presents results regarding relative frequency of different NTM species among populations with NTM disease.

In the Baixada Santista region of São Paolo, Brazil, investigators reported on a series of patients who, as patients with suspected or presumed TB, had sputum collected in regional

Table 4
Age and sex distribution of NTM lung disease by region

Location (Dates)	N	Mean Age (y)	Female (%)	COPD (%)	Preexisting Pulmonary Disease (%)
North America					
New York City, USA single institution (2000–2004)[79]	81	70	Overall 60	NR	44
Oregon, USA, statewide population based (2005–2006)[34]	407	68 (median)	60.5	NR	NR
Portland, Oregon, USA (2005–2006)[4]	134	(Subset of statewide study)	(Subset of statewide study)	28	NR
Ontario, Canada, population based (2008; MAC only)[85]	880	69.1 (median)	56	NR	NR
Toronto, Canada, single institution (2002–2003)[37]	255	68	55	39	56
Charlottesville, Virginia, USA, single institution (2001–2009)[38]	83	59	66	23	NR
Europe					
Croatia, nationwide (2006–2010)[51]	167	66 (median)	44.9	NR	NR
France, multisite (2001–2003)[45]	263	Overall 64.5 MAC 70 M xenopi 60 M kansasii 54 RGM 62	Overall 46.9 MAC 60.2 M xenopi 22.7 M kansasii 20.6 RGM 68.8		Overall 54.8 MAC 71.2 M xenopi 42.4 M kansasii 20.6 RGM 50
Netherlands, nationwide (1999–2005, M xenopi)[86]	25	M xenopi 60	M xenopi 24	M xenopi 68	M xenopi 84
Croatia, nationwide (1980–2005, M xenopi)[52]	24	M xenopi 61.7	M xenopi 10	M xenopi 90	
Central Greece (2004–2006)[47]	16	66.1	31.3	68.8	
Nijmegen-Arnhem region, Netherlands (1999–2005)[48]	53	57	30	43	70
Netherlands, nationwide (1999–2004, M chelonae-abscessus)[87]	16[a]	Overall[b] 60.2 M abscessus[a] 60.8 M chelonae 59.6	Overall[b] 25 M abscessus[a] 25 M chelonae 25	Overall 37.5 M abscessus[a] 37.5 M chelonae 37.5	Overall 62.5 M abscessus[a] 62.5 M chelonae 62.5
Denmark, nationwide (1997–2008)[5]	335	61.2	41.2	37.3	46
London, England, single institution (2000–2007, slowly growing NTM)[82]	57	61	32	37	
Netherlands, nationwide (2002–2005, M malmoense)[88]	32	M malmoense 56	M malmoense 34.4	M malmoense 66	M malmoense 81
Naples, Italy (2006–2009)[81]	16	67.6	31.3	31.3	NR
Lisbon, Portugal (2008–2009)[80]	58	Overall 54.7 (median) MAC 54.2 (median)	Overall 53.4 MAC 53.8	NR	NR

Abbreviations: MAC, *Mycobacterium avium* complex; NR, not reported; RGM, rapidly growing nontuberculous mycobacteria.

[a] Includes *M abscessus, M massiliense, M bolletii.*

[b] Patients with known cystic fibrosis excluded from above (calculated from data presented).

health care facilities, and sent to their institution for culture over the period 2000 to 2005.[39] Based on contemporary population data, their report suggests an annual prevalence of 1.3/100,000 for NTM isolation and 0.25/100,000 for NTM disease, and a 6-year period prevalence of disease of 1.5/100,000. Limitations include sampling that was not comprehensive (underestimating true rates), and disease definition based on microbiological criteria alone, perhaps overestimating the proportion with disease. From 1996 to 2005 in São Jose do Rio Preto, Brazil, investigators reported on pulmonary NTM isolation in 184 patients whose specimens had been referred to a regional TB laboratory for suspected or presumed TB.[40] Based on contemporary population data, their report suggests annual prevalence rates of 5.3/100,000 for NTM isolation and 1.0/100,000 for NTM disease, and a 10-year period prevalence of 10/100,000 for NTM disease. This report lacked information regarding the underlying sampling. If the survey was not comprehensive, the calculated rates are underestimates.

Species distribution was presented in some recent studies. In Argentina, among 54 patients with NTM PD over the period 2004 to 2010, whose specimens were submitted to a regional specialty hospital, the species distribution was MAC first (48%), followed by M kansasii (13%) and M gordonae (13%).[41] The species distribution may not apply to the entire region, depending on possible referral biases, which were not addressed. From a national mycobacterial referral center in Rio de Janeiro, Brazil, 174 patients with pulmonary NTM during 1993 through 2011 were described.[42] Because TB is generally diagnosed based on smear microscopy rather than culture, 79% of patients had been treated empirically for up to 6 months for TB before the diagnosis of NTM was made. NTM disease, defined by ATS criteria, was diagnosed in 73% (127 of 174). Among patients with NTM disease, species distribution was MAC first (35.4%), followed closely by M kansasii (33.1%), then M abscessus (18.9%), and M fortuitum (8.7%). It is uncertain whether the species distribution is regionally representative, because the report came from a highly specialized referral center, where one would suspect greater disease severity or complexity.

The finding that a large proportion of patients was initially receiving empiric, sometimes prolonged TB therapy, is consistent with the notion that NTM is likely underrecognized in regions with substantial TB rates, particularly in much of the world where laboratory capacity is not sufficient to perform cultures for the diagnosis of all patients with suspected TB. According to a report from the Para state of Brazil regarding patients with pulmonary NTM isolated from 2010 to 2011,[43] species distribution among the 29 patients who fulfilled ATS disease criteria was Mycobacterium massiliense first (44.8%), followed by MAC (20.7%), then M abscessus (6.9%). Of all positive mycobacterial cultures, 13.5% were NTM, suggesting underrecognition of NTM among TB suspects when there is exclusive reliance on smear microscopy.

Regarding population patterns, 2 recent South American studies presented data on age and sex distribution in NTM PD. Among 173 patients with NTM PD at a national mycobacterial referral center in Rio de Janeiro, Brazil, during 1993 to 2011, 62% were male and the median age was 55 years.[42] Among 29 patients with NTM PD in the Para state of Brazil with NTM PD during 2010 to 2011, 72% were female and the mean age was 52.3 years.[43] The presence of preexisting lung disease was addressed to some extent. In the study from Rio de Janeiro, bronchiectasis and COPD were present in 22% and 21% of patients, respectively, suggesting strong associations with NTM PD.[42] In the study from Para, 76% (22 of 29) of cases were thought to have prior TB.[43] On the one hand, it is plausible that bronchiectasis or other structural lung disease after TB was a major risk factor in these patients. On the other hand, the designation of prior TB was likely made without mycobacterial culture, so it is possible that at least some of the patients had NTM lung disease from the outset.

In summary, relatively little can be concluded regarding the population frequency of pulmonary NTM in Central and South America. Two studies provide data that could be used for such estimates, but the lack of a reliable population denominator makes the estimates questionable. Regional variation in the species distribution was evident among studies of NTM disease. MAC was generally most common, and M kansasii was also frequently reported. Owing to the possibility of bias in case ascertainment, it is difficult to make conclusions regarding age and sex distributions from these 2 studies.

Europe

In the European region, numerous recent studies exist using variable methodologies to study NTM epidemiology; some are population based while others use sentinel-site methods to extrapolate disease frequency over a larger region. **Table 2** presents the results of studies with data on NTM frequency while **Table 3** presents results regarding relative frequency of different NTM species among populations with NTM disease. In southwest Ireland, a population-based study of pulmonary NTM reported average annual rates of 1.9/100,000 (isolation) and 0.2/100,000 (disease) from 1987 to 2000.[44] Temporal frequency data were presented, but not by anatomic site, so inferences regarding temporal trends of pulmonary NTM could not be made.

Studies from France have used a sentinel-site methodology, collecting data over the period 2000 to 2003 from 32 sites widely distributed across the country.[31,45] Average annual rates of lung disease in patients without human immunodeficiency virus (HIV) infection were estimated for all NTM at 0.73/100,000[45] and for MAC at 0.2/100,000.[31] Estimates from these sentinel-site studies depended on several assumptions, introducing some uncertainty. The network of sentinel sites was established to provide surveillance of TB drug resistance, and prevalence estimates for NTM depend on the assumption that the population serviced by the network is identical for TB and NTM, with identical referral patterns into the network for TB and NTM. If referral into the network is not comprehensive, perhaps affected by regional providers' perception of network sites' interest or expertise, results from sentinel sites may not be appropriately generalized to the entire population.

Data from Leeds, United Kingdom, from 1995 to 1999 indicated an annual rate of NTM isolation of approximately 2.9/100,000 and disease of 1.7/100,000.[46] In Central Greece, from 2004 to 2006, annual rates of pulmonary NTM were 7.0/100,000 (isolation) and 0.7/100,000 (disease).[47] The Nijmegen-Arnhem region of the Netherlands has been extensively studied. Investigators reported annual isolation of approximately 6.3/100,000 and disease of approximately 1.4/100,000, over the period 1999 to 2005.[48] Detailed analysis of NTM epidemiology throughout Denmark from 1997 to 2008 revealed rates of average annual isolation of 2.5/100,000 and disease of 1.1/100,000.[5] Period prevalence was not presented, but a crude approximation, based on the reported median survival of approximately 5 years, is 5 to 8 per 100,000. A population-based study from Crete, Greece conducted from 2000 to 2009 reported an annual rate of disease of 0.6/100,000.[49] In the Borders region of Scotland, from 1992 to 2010, the average annual rate of NTM lung disease was reported as 1.6/100,000.[50] In Croatia, from 2006 to 2010, the annual rates of NTM isolation and disease (based on ATS microbiological criteria) were observed to be 5.3/100,000 and 0.75/100,000, respectively.[51]

Temporal trends in pulmonary NTM were presented, to some extent, in 4 studies. There was a suggestion of a temporal increase in NTM PD in Leeds, United Kingdom, over the period 1995 to 1999, although the observed absolute prevalence rates were low.[46] In Croatia, the annual identification of M xenopi pulmonary disease increased steadily from 0.05/100,000 from the early 1980s to 0.18/100,000 in the early 2000s.[52] Data from the national reference laboratory for mycobacteria in the Netherlands (receiving 85% of clinically isolated NTM) from 2000 to 2006 demonstrated an approximate 4-fold increase in the number of patients referred with M avium isolates.[53] Although changes in referral rates could explain some of the increase, there was likely a substantial increase in pulmonary M avium. In the Scottish Borders region, from 1992 to 2010, there was a substantial increase in NTM lung disease, from 0.86/100,000 in 1992-2004 to 3.1/100,000 in 2005-2010.[50]

Several European studies have presented useful data regarding age, sex, and preexisting lung disease in NTM PD (see **Table 4**). The following weighted mean calculations were performed among studies presented in **Table 4** with nonoverlapping populations. There was an average age of approximately 62.5 years, apparently somewhat younger than the mean age of NTM PD patients in North American studies. All but one study reported that patients were mostly men (mean 57%), in contrast to findings in North America. The presence of COPD, when reported, was described in 39% of NTM PD patients.

In summary, recent literature from Europe continues to identify substantially lower rates of pulmonary NTM isolation and disease than in North America, with several studies demonstrating recent temporal increases. In contrast to observations in North America, NTM PD patients in European studies tend be mostly men, and slightly younger. Some of the differences likely relate to differences in smoking patterns. Recent data suggest that in Europe, 23% of adults are smokers (with a 16% reduction during the prior decade), whereas in the United States and Canada, approximately 15% of adults are smokers (with a 16% reduction during the prior decade). Based on differences in recent smoking data, one might assume that a higher proportion of NTM PD in Europe would be COPD/smoking-related,[54] and, perhaps because of a historical excess of men smoking, that men would comprise a higher proportion of NTM PD patients.

Africa

Numerous recent African studies have investigated the frequency of pulmonary NTM in 2 main types of populations. First, several investigations searched for NTM among patients suspected of having pulmonary TB. In 10 hospitals in western Kenya, from 2007 to 2009, 361 of 872 (45.1%) patients suspected of having pulmonary TB tested positive for mycobacteria. Of patients with positive cultures, 95.8% (346 of 361) had TB while 4.2% (15 of 361) had NTM.[55] In 2 TB centers in Nigeria, during 2010 and 2011, consecutive TB suspects were assessed with mycobacterial cultures in addition to acid-fast bacilli (AFB) smear.[56] Of 1603 TB suspects, 444 (28%) had pulmonary mycobacteria identified, of whom 375 (85%) had *Mycobacterium tuberculosis* complex species and 69 (15%) had NTM.[56] Finally, in a surveillance study of children and adolescents in rural Eastern Uganda, including 2200 individuals identified as pulmonary TB suspects, only 8 patients (0.36%) had *M tuberculosis* complex species isolated, whereas 95 patients (4.3%) had NTM isolated.[57] Although these studies did not provide adequate details regarding the proportion of patients who fulfilled criteria for NTM disease, the results suggest that a potentially significant proportion of African TB suspects may have NTM disease but may not be detected in routine care.

The second relevant population type that has been studied comprises patients with "chronic" pulmonary TB. In Burkina Faso, from 2007 to 2008, patients classified as having chronic TB (positive acid-fast sputum smear after 5 months of standard therapy) were investigated microbiologically to assess the common assumption that chronic TB accurately identifies multidrug-resistant (MDR) TB.[58] Of 63 cases investigated, 38 patients (60.3%) had *M tuberculosis* complex species isolated while 13 (20.6%) had NTM. In a similar study from a TB referral center in Mali, 61 chronic TB patients were investigated, of whom 11 (18%) were found to have only NTM in their sputum.[59] These findings suggest that a substantial proportion of patients in Africa with suspected MDR TB may actually have NTM PD.

Middle East and South Asia

No recent population-based studies of pulmonary NTM were identified from this region. Several studies, generally performed in single institutions, provide information regarding species distribution among patients with NTM PD in this region. At a single center in Turkey, during 2004 to 2009, among 53 patients with pulmonary NTM isolation, 60% (31 of 53) were judged to have disease.[60] The mean age of patients with disease was 54 years, 87.1% (27 of 31) of whom were male.[60] In a single institution in Israel, among 215 patients identified with pulmonary NTM isolation over the period

2004 to 2010, 21% (45 of 215) were judged to have definite or probable disease, but clinical information was not detailed.[61] From various laboratories in Saudi Arabia, a sample of 95 patients with NTM isolation was identified during 2009 and 2010, including 73 patients with pulmonary isolation, 67% of whom (49 of 73) were judged to have pulmonary disease, but clinical information was not detailed.[62] In Oman, from 2006 to 2007, a random sample of 13 NTM isolates from the Central Public Health Laboratory in Muscat was selected for case review.[63] Eleven isolates were pulmonary, and ATS disease criteria were fulfilled in 63.6% (7 of 11). Among patients with NTM PD the mean age was 46.3 years, and 57.1% (4 of 7) were male. At a single institution in Mumbai, India, during 2005 to 2008, 103 patients had pulmonary NTM isolates, with 65.0% (67 of 103) judged to have either "definite" or "probable" disease, but clinical information was not detailed.[64] **Table 3** presents the species distributions among patients with NTM PD from the aforementioned studies.

East Asia

No population-based studies of pulmonary NTM epidemiology in East Asia were identified. Several studies from single institutions have been published, and are described herein. Generally excluded are studies that presented exclusively isolate-level data (lacking patient-level data) and studies that focused on specific patient groups (critical care unit patients, cancer patients, and so forth). Several South Korean studies offer insight into NTM PD species distribution and patient characteristics, and suggest that NTM PD is becoming increasingly common. At one institution in Seoul during 2002 and 2003, 794 patients with pulmonary NTM isolates were classified according to disease status[65] using the 1997 ATS criteria[66] and the 2000 British Thoracic Society (BTS) criteria,[67] ascertained by full review of medical records.[65] Definite disease was defined by fulfilling both ATS and BTS criteria, probable disease cases fulfilled only the BTS (less stringent) criteria, and unlikely disease comprised the remainder. Of 195 patients judged to have either definite (n = 131) or possible (n = 64) disease, the mean age was 63 years, and 55% were women. The species distribution is shown in **Table 3**.

Recent Japanese studies provide insight into the prevalence of NTM PD, species distribution, and patient features. A recent study used the mortality rate among patients with NTM PD as a way to derive estimates of prevalence of NTM PD.[10] The investigators estimated a national prevalence of NTM PD in Japan in 2005 at 33 to 65 per

100,000, and reported that most cases are caused by MAC.[10] A single-institution study in Tokyo, describing 273 newly diagnosed patients with MAC lung disease during 1996 to 2002, reported an average age of 64 years and a predominance of females (70%).[68] The investigators divided the disease into radiographic type according to the presence of cavitation, and observed that 30% of females had cavitation, compared with 65% to 70% of males. Two additional studies of MAC PD patients from Japan provide interesting insights.[69,70] Among 634 HIV-negative patients diagnosed with MAC PD from 1995 to 2005 in Saitama, the mean age at cohort entry was 68.9 years, 58.5% were women, and 38.3% had preexisting respiratory disease (including 5.8% with emphysema).[69] Another group presented data on a cohort of 164 patients identified with MAC PD from 1999 to 2005 in Kyoto, wherein the mean age was 66 years, 56.7% were women, and 61.6% had COPD.[70] These studies support the notion that MAC PD patients in Japan are generally older and mostly women, although the presence of COPD is variable. However, referral bias may affect cohort characteristics in studies from single institutions.

Several studies from single institutions in Taiwan provide insights into species distribution and suggest that NTM PD is increasingly common. At an institution in Kaohsiung City, southern Taiwan, it was observed during 2004 and 2005 that among the 67 patients with NTM PD identified, the average age was 67 years, 70% were male, and 88.1% had preexisting lung disease including 61.2% with COPD.[71] At a hospital in Taipei City, northern Taiwan, the annual prevalence of NTM PD increased from 1.28/100,000 in 2000 to 7.94/100,000 in 2008.[72] From the same institution, 252 NTM PD patients with classifiable radiographic patterns (cavitary, bronchiectatic, or consolidative) were identified over the period 2007 to 2009.[73] The mean age was 63.7 years, and 50.8% were men.[73] The studies from Taiwan identified NTM PD patients as being in the same age range as reported in most other studies. However, in contrast to work from Japan and Korea, Taiwanese studies described a slight male predominance. Referral biases may be relevant in these single-institution studies. Species distribution data from these studies are presented in **Table 3**.

Two recent studies from China reported on the frequency of NTM isolation among patients with mycobacterial isolates. In a single institution in Shanghai over the period 2005 to 2008, 5.1% of positive mycobacterial cultures were NTM, increasing from 4.3% in 2005 to 6.4% in 2008.[74] In several counties in rural Shandong Province,

of 2949 specimens that were culture-positive for mycobacteria, 64 were NTM (1.6%).[75] More detailed epidemiologic data from China are not yet readily available.

In summary, recent NTM PD studies from East Asia describe patients who are usually in their seventh decade (mean/median age 63–69 years). South Korean and Japanese investigators identified mostly females, whereas Taiwanese research reported a slight male predominance.

Australia and New Zealand

Recent literature from Australia and New Zealand includes 3 excellent population-based studies describing the epidemiology of NTM PD. **Table 2** presents data regarding disease frequency while **Table 3** presents data regarding NTM species distribution. A nationwide Australian survey during 2000, focusing on incidence (patients without previously identified pulmonary NTM), reported an annual isolation incidence of 5.9/100,000 and disease incidence of 0.56/100,000.[76] In the state of Queensland, Australia, data were presented from 1999 to 2005. In the most recent year of study, the annual prevalence of NTM PD was 3.2/100,000.[2] In New Zealand, in 2004 it was observed that the prevalence of NTM PD was 1.17/100,000.[77] Temporal trends in NTM PD were presented in 2 Australian studies. At the nationwide level, comparing 2000 with 1988, there appeared to be a minimal increase in annual incidence, from 0.51/100,000 to 0.56/100,000.[76] In Queensland, there was an increase from 2.2/100,000 to 3.2/100,000 from 1999 to 2005.[2] In the latter study, note was made of a predominance of fibronodular (nodular bronchiectatic) disease in the most recent year of the study, compared with a previously reported predominance of cavitary disease.

Regarding age and sex distributions, in Queensland, appreciable rates of NTM PD occurred among patients who were at least 45 years old and increased dramatically with age, with a tripling in rates between the 45- to 59-year-old age group and the 60- to 74-year-old age group.[2] In addition, women outnumbered men overall and in all age strata from 30 years and older. In New Zealand, 79% of people with NTM PD were female, but age data were not presented.[77] Also in New Zealand, 82% of NTM PD patients were described as having predisposing lung conditions, including 18% with COPD and 56% with bronchiectasis, whereby cause versus effect may be difficult to discern.[77]

SUMMARY AND RESEARCH GAPS

Population-based data for prevalence and trends estimation are available primarily from North

America, Europe, and New Zealand and Australia, where NTM PD is a reportable condition; these data have documented a continued increase in NTM prevalence since 2000. Annual prevalence in North America and Australia, ranging from 3.2 to 9.8, is generally higher than in Europe, where available estimates are all below 2 per 100,000. Tertiary care–based studies of NTM PD from South Korea, Japan, and Taiwan also suggest increasing prevalence of NTM PD. In South America, Africa, and the Middle East, studies among patients with suspected TB and MDR have documented a previously unappreciated prevalence of NTM in this population, ranging from 4% to 15% for suspected TB and 18% to 20% for suspected MDR TB.

Clinical data available from several regions have allowed better characterization of the affected populations. Across regions, most cases occur among persons older than 50 years, with a mean age of 54 to 70 years. In North America and East Asia, most NTM PD cases are among women, whereas in Europe men predominate among NTM PD cases, with varying proportions of preexisting lung disease across regions. The species distribution also varies by region, with MAC predominant in North America and East Asia, whereas in Europe MAC is less predominant and *M kansasii*, *M xenopi*, and *Mycobacterium malmoense* are found with greater frequency. In addition, species vary by patients' sex and the presence of preexisting lung disease.

The available data highlight data needs and research gaps. To more fully characterize prevalence and trends for NTM PD, population-based data on NTM isolates with species information linked to clinical data and patient characteristics (age, sex, geographic location) are needed from more geographic areas of the world. These data could be obtained by linking NTM surveillance to existing TB surveillance, with reporting of all AFB isolates linked to this clinical and demographic information. In areas where such data are not feasible to obtain, sentinel surveillance could be established at tertiary care centers serving a large population. In particular, to advance the understanding of the influence of species and subspecies type on disease type and progression, in addition to the influence of environmental reservoirs on disease presentation, more detailed information related to both patient and demographic factors are needed. Standard microbiological and clinical data collection will allow assessment of trends. The detection of important proportions of patients with NTM isolates among patients screened for TB and MDR TB highlights the need for enhanced mycobacterial laboratory capacity to discriminate between cases of TB and NTM, ensuring correct diagnosis and management, and the identification of the burden of NTM in these settings.

With respect to risk factors for NTM, host and environmental factors interact to influence disease risk. Beyond previously described structural abnormalities and immunosuppressive conditions, host factors important to the current epidemiology of NTM PD include thoracic skeletal abnormalities, rheumatoid arthritis, immunomodulatory drugs such as tumor necrosis factor α inhibitors (particularly in the rheumatoid arthritis population), steroid use, and gastrointestinal reflux disease. Clustering of disease within families suggests a heritable genetic predisposition to disease and additional research is needed to identify these genetic factors. With respect to environmental exposures to water and soil aerosols, very few individual exposures have been identified, but new analytical approaches have highlighted the importance of climatic factors, such as warm, humid environments with high atmospheric vapor pressure, as contributing to population risk. Further research is needed to more specifically identify additional climatic and soil factors and their contribution to microbial growth. Furthermore, the interaction of human populations with these environments will be key to understanding the interaction of host and environmental factors.

ACKNOWLEDGMENTS

This work was supported in part by the Division of Intramural Research, National Institutes of Allergy and Infectious Diseases, National Institutes of Health. We would also like to acknowledge Ms. Sara Strollo for her assistance with manuscript preparation.

REFERENCES

1. Marras TK, Daley CL. Epidemiology of human pulmonary infection with nontuberculous mycobacteria. Clin Chest Med 2002;23:553–67.
2. Thomson RM, NTM working group at Queensland TB Control Centre and Queensland Mycobacterial Reference Laboratory. Changing epidemiology of pulmonary nontuberculous mycobacteria infections. Emerg Infect Dis 2010;16:1576–83.
3. Prevots DR, Shaw PA, Strickland D, et al. Nontuberculous mycobacterial lung disease prevalence at four integrated health care delivery systems. Am J Respir Crit Care Med 2010;182:970–6.
4. Winthrop KL, McNelley E, Kendall B, et al. Pulmonary nontuberculous mycobacterial disease prevalence and clinical features: an emerging public

health disease. Am J Respir Crit Care Med 2010; 182:977–82.

5. Andrejak C, Thomsen VO, Johansen IS, et al. Nontuberculous pulmonary mycobacteriosis in Denmark: incidence and prognostic factors. Am J Respir Crit Care Med 2010;181:514–21.

6. Griffith DE, Aksamit T, Brown-Elliott BA, et al. An official ATS/IDSA statement: diagnosis, treatment, and prevention of nontuberculous mycobacterial diseases. Am J Respir Crit Care Med 2007;175:367–416.

7. Adjemian J, Olivier KN, Seitz AE, et al. Prevalence of nontuberculous mycobacterial lung disease in U.S. Medicare beneficiaries. Am J Respir Crit Care Med 2012;185:881–6.

8. Marras TK, Mendelson D, Marchand-Austin A, et al. Pulmonary nontuberculous mycobacterial disease, Ontario, Canada, 1998-2010. Emerg Infect Dis 2013;19:1889–91.

9. Mirsaeidi M, Machado RF, Garcia JG, et al. Nontuberculous mycobacterial disease mortality in the United States, 1999-2010: a population-based comparative study. PLoS One 2014;9:e91879.

10. Morimoto K, Iwai K, Uchimura K, et al. A steady increase in nontuberculous mycobacteriosis mortality and estimated prevalence in Japan. Ann Am Thorac Soc 2014;11:1–8.

11. Colombo RE, Hill SC, Claypool RJ, et al. Familial clustering of pulmonary nontuberculous mycobacterial disease. Chest 2010;137:629–34.

12. Leung JM, Fowler C, Smith C, et al. A familial syndrome of pulmonary nontuberculous mycobacteria infections. Am J Respir Crit Care Med 2013;188: 1373–6.

13. Cutting GR. Modifier genes in mendelian disorders: the example of cystic fibrosis. Ann N Y Acad Sci 2010;1214:57–69.

14. Kubo K, Yamazaki Y, Hanaoka M, et al. Analysis of HLA antigens in *Mycobacterium avium-intracellulare* pulmonary infection. Am J Respir Crit Care Med 2000;161:1368–71.

15. Takahashi M, Ishizaka A, Nakamura H, et al. Specific HLA in pulmonary MAC infection in a Japanese population. Am J Respir Crit Care Med 2000;162:316–8.

16. Feazel LM, Baumgartner LK, Peterson KL, et al. Opportunistic pathogens enriched in showerhead biofilms. Proc Natl Acad Sci U S A 2009;106: 16393–9.

17. Adjemian J, Olivier KN, Seitz AE, et al. Spatial clusters of nontuberculous mycobacterial lung disease in the United States. Am J Respir Crit Care Med 2012;186:553–8.

18. Chou MP, Clements AC, Thomson RM. A spatial epidemiological analysis of nontuberculous mycobacterial infections in Queensland, Australia. BMC Infect Dis 2014;14:279.

19. Dirac MA, Horan KL, Doody DR, et al. Environment or host?: A case-control study of risk factors for *Mycobacterium avium* complex lung disease. Am J Respir Crit Care Med 2012;186:684–91.

20. Prevots DR, Adjemian J, Fernandez AG, et al. Environmental risks for nontuberculous mycobacteria: individual exposures and climatic factors in the cystic fibrosis population. Ann Am Thorac Soc 2014;11:1032–8.

21. Maekawa K, Ito Y, Hirai T, et al. Environmental risk factors for pulmonary mycobacterium avium-intracellulare complex disease. Chest 2011;140: 723–9.

22. Olivier KN, Weber DJ, Wallace RJ Jr, et al. Nontuberculous mycobacteria. I: multicenter prevalence study in cystic fibrosis. Am J Respir Crit Care Med 2003;167:828–34.

23. Andrejak C, Nielsen R, Thomsen VO, et al. Chronic respiratory disease, inhaled corticosteroids and risk of non-tuberculous mycobacteriosis. Thorax 2013;68: 256–62.

24. Prince DS, Peterson DD, Steiner RM, et al. Infection with *Mycobacterium avium* complex in patients without predisposing conditions. N Engl J Med 1989;321:863–8.

25. Kim RD, Greenberg DE, Ehrmantraut ME, et al. Pulmonary nontuberculous mycobacterial disease: prospective study of a distinct preexisting syndrome. Am J Respir Crit Care Med 2008;178:1066–74.

26. Brode SK, Jamieson FB, Ng R, et al. Risk of mycobacterial infections associated with rheumatoid arthritis in Ontario, Canada. Chest 2014;146:563–72.

27. Winthrop KL, Baxter R, Liu L, et al. Mycobacterial diseases and antitumour necrosis factor therapy in USA. Ann Rheum Dis 2013;72:37–42.

28. Adjemian J, Olivier KN, Prevots DR. Nontuberculous mycobacteria among cystic fibrosis patients in the United States: screening practices and environmental risk. Am J Respir Crit Care Med 2014; 190:581–6.

29. Edwards LB, Acquaviva FA, Livesay VT, et al. Clinical and laboratory studies of tuberculosis and respiratory disease: the Navy Recruit Program. Am Rev Respir Dis 1969;99:1–132.

30. Kirschner RA Jr, Parker BC, Falkinham JO III. Epidemiology of infection by nontuberculous mycobacteria. *Mycobacterium avium*, *Mycobacterium intracellulare*, and *Mycobacterium scrofulaceum* in acid, brown-water swamps of the southeastern United States and their association with environmental variables. Am Rev Respir Dis 1992;145: 271–5.

31. Maugein J, Dailloux M, Carbonelle B, et al. Sentinel site surveillance of *Mycobacterium avium* complex pulmonary disease. Eur Respir J 2005;26:1092–6.

32. Winthrop KL, Baxter R, Liu L, et al. The reliability of diagnostic coding and laboratory data to identify tuberculosis and nontuberculous mycobacterial disease among rheumatoid arthritis patients using

anti-tumor necrosis factor therapy. Pharmacoepide-miol Drug Saf 2011;20:229–35.

33. Hoefsloot W, van Ingen J, Andrejak C, et al. The geographic diversity of nontuberculous mycobacte-ria isolated from pulmonary samples: an NTM-NET collaborative study. Eur Respir J 2013;42:1604–13.

34. Cassidy PM, Hedberg K, Saulson A, et al. Nontuber-culous mycobacterial disease prevalence and risk factors: a changing epidemiology. Clin Infect Dis 2009;49:e124–9.

35. Marras TK, Chedore P, Ying AM, et al. Isolation prev-alence of pulmonary non-tuberculous mycobacteria in Ontario 1997-2003. Thorax 2007;62:661–6.

36. Al-Houqani M, Jamieson F, Chedore P, et al. Isola-tion prevalence of pulmonary nontuberculous mycobacteria in Ontario in 2007. Can Respir J 2011;18:19–24.

37. Marras TK, Mehta M, Chedore P, et al. Nontuber-culous mycobacterial lung infections in Ontario, Can-ada: clinical and microbiological characteristics. Lung 2010;188:289–99.

38. Satyanarayana G, Heysell SK, Scully KW, et al. Mycobacterial infections in a large Virginia hospital, 2001-2009. BMC Infect Dis 2011;11:113.

39. Zamarioli LA, Coelho AG, Pereira CM, et al. Descriptive study of the frequency of nontubercu-lous mycobacteria in the Baixada Santista region of the state of Sao Paulo, Brazil. J Bras Pneumol 2008;34:590–4.

40. Pedro HS, Pereira MI, Goloni MR, et al. Nontubercu-lous mycobacteria isolated in Sao Jose do Rio Preto, Brazil between 1996 and 2005. J Bras Pneumol 2008;34:950–5.

41. Imperiale B, Zumarraga M, Gioffre A, et al. Disease caused by non-tuberculous mycobacteria: diag-nostic procedures and treatment evaluation in the north of Buenos Aires Province. Rev Argent Micro-biol 2012;44:3–9.

42. de Mello KG, Mello FC, Borga L, et al. Clinical and therapeutic features of pulmonary nontuberculous mycobacterial disease, Brazil, 1993-2011. Emerg Infect Dis 2013;19:393–9.

43. Fusco da Costa AR, Falkinham JO III, Lopes ML, et al. Occurrence of nontuberculous mycobacterial pulmonary infection in an endemic area of tubercu-losis. PLoS Negl Trop Dis 2013;7:e2340 [Electronic resource].

44. Kennedy MP, O'Connor TM, Ryan C, et al. Nontuber-culous mycobacteria: incidence in Southwest Ireland from 1987 to 2000. Respir Med 2003;97:257–63.

45. Dailloux M, Abalain ML, Laurain C, et al. Respiratory infections associated with nontuberculous myco-bacteria in non-HIV patients. Eur Respir J 2006;28:1211–5.

46. Henry MT, Inamdar L, O'Riordain D, et al. Nontuber-culous mycobacteria in non-HIV patients: epidemiology, treatment and response. Eur Respir J 2004;23:741–6.

47. Gerogianni I, Papala M, Kostikas K, et al. Epidemi-ology and clinical significance of mycobacterial res-piratory infections in Central Greece. Int J Tuberc Lung Dis 2008;12:807–12.

48. Van Ingen J, Bendien SA, de Lange WC, et al. Clinical relevance of nontuberculous mycobacteria isolated in Nijmegen-Arnhem region, The Netherlands. Thorax 2009;64:502–6.

49. Gitti Z, Mantadakis E, Maraki S, et al. Clinical signif-icance and antibiotic susceptibilities of nontubercu-lous mycobacteria from patients in Crete, Greece. Future Microbiol 2011;6:1099–109.

50. McCallum AD, Watkin SW, Faccenda JF. Non-tuber-culous mycobacterial infections in the Scottish Bor-ders: identification, management and treatment outcomes–a retrospective review. J R Coll Physicians Edinb 2011;41:294–303.

51. Jankovic M, Samarzija M, Sabol I, et al. Geographical distribution and clinical relevance of non-tuberculous mycobacteria in Croatia. Int J Tuberc Lung Dis 2013;17:836–41.

52. Marusic A, Katalinic-Jankovic V, Popovic-Grle S, et al. Mycobacterium xenopi pulmonary dis-ease—epidemiology and clinical features in non-immunocompromised patients. J Infect 2009;58:108–12.

53. van Ingen J, Hoefsloot W, Dekhuijzen PN, et al. The changing pattern of clinical Mycobacterium avium isolation in the Netherlands. Int J Tuberc Lung Dis 2010;14:1176–80.

54. OECD. OECD factbook 2014: economic, environ-mental and social statistics. OECD Publishing; 2014. Available at: http://www.oecd-ilibrary.org/economics/oecd-factbook-2014_factbook-2014-en. Accesssed October 29, 2014.

55. Nyamogoba HD, Mbuthia G, Mining S, et al. HIV co-infection with tuberculous and non-tuberculous mycobacteria in western Kenya: challenges in the diagnosis and management. Afr Health Sci 2012;12:305–11.

56. Aliyu G, El-Kamary SS, Abimiku A, et al. Prevalence of non-tuberculous mycobacterial infections among tuberculosis suspects in Nigeria. PLoS One 2013;8:e63170 [Electronic resource].

57. Asiimwe BB, Bagyenzi GB, Ssengooba W, et al. Species and genotypic diversity of non-tuberculous mycobacteria isolated from children investigated for pulmonary tuberculosis in rural Uganda. BMC Infect Dis 2013;13:88.

58. Badoum G, Saleri N, Dembele MS, et al. Failing a re-treatment regimen does not predict MDR/XDR tuberculosis: is "blind" treatment dangerous? Eur Respir J 2011;37:1283–5.

59. Maiga M, Siddiqui S, Diallo S, et al. Failure to recog-nize nontuberculous mycobacteria leads to misdiag-nosis of chronic pulmonary tuberculosis. PLoS One 2012;7:e36902 [Electronic resource].

60. Bicmen C, Coskun M, Gunduz AT, et al. Nontuberculous mycobacteria isolated from pulmonary specimens between 2004 and 2009: causative agent or not? New Microbiol 2010;33:399–403.

61. Braun E, Sprecher H, Davidson S, et al. Epidemiology and clinical significance of non-tuberculous mycobacteria isolated from pulmonary specimens. Int J Tuberc Lung Dis 2012;17:96–9.

62. Varghese B, Memish Z, Abuljadayel N, et al. Emergence of clinically relevant non-tuberculous mycobacterial infections in Saudi Arabia. PLoS Negl Trop Dis 2013;7:e2234 [Electronic resource].

63. Al-Mahruqi SH, van-Ingen J, Al-Busaidy S, et al. Clinical relevance of nontuberculous mycobacteria, Oman. Emerg Infect Dis 2009;15:292–4.

64. Shenai S, Rodrigues C, Mehta A. Time to identify and define non-tuberculous mycobacteria in a tuberculosis-endemic region. Int J Tuberc Lung Dis 2010;14:1001–8.

65. Koh WJ, Kwon OJ, Jeon K, et al. Clinical significance of nontuberculous mycobacteria isolated from respiratory specimens in Korea. Chest 2006; 129:341–8.

66. American Thoracic Society. Diagnosis and treatment of disease caused by nontuberculous mycobacteria. Am J Respir Crit Care Med 1997;156: S1–25.

67. British Thoracic Society. Management of opportunist mycobacterial infections: Joint tuberculosis committee guidelines 1999. Thorax 2000;55:210–8.

68. Okumura M, Iwai K, Ogata H, et al. Clinical factors on cavitary and nodular bronchiectatic types in pulmonary *Mycobacterium avium* complex disease. Intern Med 2008;47:1465–72.

69. Hayashi M, Takayanagi N, Kanauchi T, et al. Prognostic factors of 634 HIV-negative patients with *Mycobacterium avium* complex lung disease. Am J Respir Crit Care Med 2012;185:575–83.

70. Ito Y, Hirai T, Maekawa K, et al. Predictors of 5-year mortality in pulmonary *Mycobacterium avium-intracellulare* complex disease. Int J Tuberc Lung Dis 2012;16:408–14.

71. Wang CC, Lin MC, Liu JW, et al. Nontuberculous mycobacterial lung disease in southern Taiwan. Chang Gung Med J 2009;32:499–508.

72. Lai CC, Tan CK, Chou CH, et al. Increasing incidence of nontuberculous mycobacteria, Taiwan, 2000-2008. Emerg Infect Dis 2010;16:294–6.

73. Shu CC, Lee CH, Hsu CL, et al. Clinical characteristics and prognosis of nontuberculous mycobacterial lung disease with different radiographic patterns. Lung 2011;189:467–74.

74. Wang HX, Yue J, Han M, et al. Nontuberculous mycobacteria: susceptibility pattern and prevalence rate in Shanghai from 2005 to 2008. Chin Med J 2010;123:184–7.

75. Jing H, Wang H, Wang Y, et al. Prevalence of nontuberculous mycobacteria infection, China, 2004-2009. Emerg Infect Dis 2012;18:527–8.

76. Haverkort F. National atypical mycobacteria survey, 2000. Commun Dis Intell Q Rep 2003;27:180–9.

77. Freeman J, Morris A, Blackmore T, et al. Incidence of nontuberculous mycobacterial disease in New Zealand, 2004. N Z Med J 2007;120:U2580.

78. Brode SK, Jamieson FB, Ng R, et al. Population-based risk of mycobacterial infections associated with anti-tumor necrosis factor (anti-TNF) therapy in older patients in Ontario, Canada. Chest 2013; 144(4_MeetingAbstracts):270A. http://dx.doi.org/10.1378/chest.1704023.

79. Bodle EE, Cunnigham JA, Della-Latta P, et al. Epidemiology of nontuberculous mycobacteria in patients without HIV infection, New York City. Emerg Infect Dis 2008;14:390–6.

80. Amorim A, Macedo R, Lopes A, et al. Non-tuberculous mycobacteria in HIV-negative patients with pulmonary disease in Lisbon, Portugal. Scand J Infect Dis 2010;42:626–8.

81. Del Giudice G, Iadevaia C, Santoro G, et al. Nontuberculous mycobacterial lung disease in patients without HIV infection: a retrospective analysis over 3 years. Clin Respir J 2011;5:203–10.

82. Davies BS, Roberts CH, Kaul S, et al. Non-tuberculous slow-growing mycobacterial pulmonary infections in non-HIV-infected patients in south London. Scand J Infect Dis 2012;44:815–9.

83. Park YS, Lee CH, Lee SM, et al. Rapid increase of non-tuberculous mycobacterial lung diseases at a tertiary referral hospital in South Korea. Int J Tuberc Lung Dis 2010;14:1069–71.

84. Lee SK, Lee EJ, Kim SK, et al. Changing epidemiology of nontuberculous mycobacterial lung disease in South Korea. Scand J Infect Dis 2012;44:733–8.

85. Al-Houqani M, Jamieson F, Mehta M, et al. Aging, COPD and other risk factors do not explain the increased prevalence of pulmonary *Mycobacterium avium* complex in Ontario. Chest 2012;141:190–7.

86. van Ingen J, Boeree MJ, de Lange WC, et al. *Mycobacterium xenopi* clinical relevance and determinants, the Netherlands. Emerg Infect Dis 2008;14: 385–9.

87. van Ingen J, de Zwaan R, Dekhuijzen RP, et al. Clinical relevance of *Mycobacterium chelonae-abscessus* group isolation in 95 patients. J Infect 2009;59: 324–31.

88. Hoefsloot W, van Ingen J, de Lange WC, et al. Clinical relevance of *Mycobacterium malmoense* isolation in The Netherlands. Eur Respir J 2009;34:926–31.

Environmental Sources of Nontuberculous Mycobacteria

Joseph O. Falkinham III, PhD

KEYWORDS

- *Mycobacterium* • Drinking water • Soil • Aerosolization

KEY POINTS

- Nontuberculous mycobacteria (NTM) are opportunistic pathogens; sources include drinking water, natural water, and soils. NTM are not contaminants, but normal inhabitants of those habitats.
- Human infection occurs because NTM are in the same habitats that humans encounter and are thereby exposed to waters, aerosols, or dusts that can be inhaled or swallowed.
- NTM are more resistant to common water disinfectants, such as chlorine, and their use selects NTM persistence in drinking water distribution systems and household plumbing.
- Because NTM patients are subject to reinfection, it is of value for water providers and homeowners to consider measures to reduce exposure to NTM.

INTRODUCTION

The nontuberculous mycobacteria (NTM) are opportunistic human pathogens that are normal inhabitants of the environment, especially the human-engineered environment. A list of those habitats in presented in **Box 1**. NTM are ideally suited for residence and growth in the habitats they share with humans, particularly plumbing in buildings, hospitals, apartment houses, and homes. Once NTM are introduced (eg, via drinking water), they attach to surfaces and grow to form a biofilm. That plumbing biofilm becomes a source of infection. Infection occurs after transmission from the environment, for example, from NTM in household shower aerosols[1] or from NTM in potting soil dusts.[2]

It is the objective of this article to identify NTM sources and routes of transmission. Such information can be used by individuals of increased susceptibility and their physicians to suggest measures to reduce exposure and thereby reduce infection or reinfection. At the outset, it is important

to point out that the majority of the data in this article have been gained by the study of *Mycobacterium avium* subspecies *hominissuis*, the predominant NTM opportunist in the United States. The lessons taught certainly hold for that *M avium* subspecies, but may not hold for other NTM species or even close relatives of *M avium*, such as *Mycobacterium intracellulare*.

NONTUBERCULOUS MYCOBACTERIA

The NTM group currently encompasses over 150 individual species.[3] All, with few exceptions, are opportunistic pathogens. The dramatic increase in new *Mycobacterium* species is owing to:

1. Increased susceptibility of individuals infected with the human immunodeficiency virus to NTM infection,
2. Improved techniques for primary culture of NTM, and
3. Detection of infection by direct DNA isolation and sequencing.

Disclosure: None.
Department of Biological Sciences, Virginia Tech, 1405 Perry Street, Blacksburg, VA 24061-0406, USA
E-mail address: jofiii@vt.edu

Clin Chest Med 36 (2015) 35–41
http://dx.doi.org/10.1016/j.ccm.2014.10.003
0272-5231/15/$ – see front matter © 2015 Elsevier Inc. All rights reserved.

Because the ecology, sources, physiology, virulence, and antibiotic susceptibility of the NTM species can differ a great deal, accurate species identification is a must. It is inadequate to designate a patient as infected with *M avium* complex or *M avium–intracellulare*. For example, *M avium* subsp. *hominissuis* is found in water, but not *M intracellulare*; its source is soil.

The NTM are particularly well-adapted to human-engineered environments, such as drinking water distribution systems and plumbing in buildings. The lipid-rich, mycolic acid–containing outer membrane of NTM result in cells that are the most hydrophobic among the bacteria.[4] Their cell surface hydrophobicity contributes to their:

- Concentration in water droplets arising from bodies of water,[5]
- Adherence to plumbing pipe surfaces,[6] and
- Broad spectrum resistance to disinfectants[7] and antibiotics.[8]

The slow growth of NTM (generally 1 generation per day at 37°C) does not reflect a slower metabolism, but the fact that a substantial amount of energy and carbon are diverted toward synthesis of the long chain fatty acids (C_{60}–C_{80}) in the outer membrane. Slow growth coupled with a rapid metabolic rate means that NTM can adapt to changing conditions (eg, starvation, antibiotic or disinfectant exposure) by inducing genes for proteins that protect cells from life-threatening conditions. NTM are also relatively resistant to the low pH encountered in the stomach.[9,10] The relative resistance of NTM to heat (50°C–60°C)[11] is also

a factor in the survival and proliferation of NTM in single family homes and apartment/condominium buildings.

SOURCES OF NONTUBERCULOUS MYCOBACTERIA

NTM are natural inhabitants of soils, lakes, rivers, and streams. **Box 1** lists NTM sources for human infection. The origin of NTM is soils, from whence it enters surface waters. Both northern hemisphere pine (boreal) forest soils[12] and southeastern US coastal acidic, brown water swamps have high numbers of NTM (10^6 per gram).[13] That habitat predilection is owing, in part, to NTM's preference for growth at acidic pH[10] and growth stimulation by humic and fulvic acids, whose concentration is high in such forest and US coastal swamp soils.[14] In addition, water draining from such forests and swamps is rich in NTM.[13,15] Such surface water is then, in turn, used as a source for drinking water. Persistence of the slowly growing NTM in rivers and streams is owing to their adherence to fixed objects, such as rocks and plant material, where they form biofilms. Because NTM are able to grow in protozoa[16] and amoebae,[17] they can survive protist grazing, unlike many other microorganisms that are part of the microbial flora. Further, it has been suggested that the ability of the NTM to grow in animal macrophages is a consequence of "training" in protozoa and amoebae. Not only is growth supported, but *M avium* cells grown in amoebae have been shown to be more virulent.[17]

From surface water sources, NTM enter drinking water treatment plants, primarily via their attachment to soil particles, based on the fact that source water turbidity reduction reduces the number of NTM entering treatment plants.[18] As a consequence of the lipid-rich outer membrane,[4] NTM are quite resistant to disinfectants, such as chlorine, chloramine, and ozone.[7] In fact, NTM are generally 40-fold more resistant to chlorine than *Pseudomonas aeruginosa* and 100-fold more resistant to chlorine than *Escherichia coli*, the standard for water treatment.[7] The death of other, disinfectant-susceptible microorganisms leaves the NTM without competition for nutrients. Coupled with the ability of the NTM to grow at low nutrient concentrations,[19] the absence of competitors, and the low concentration of disinfection in the water leaving the treatment plant, unrestricted growth of NTM can occur in the distribution system. Even when found, they are in low numbers. NTM numbers increase 2-fold in a drinking water distribution system from the treatment plant to the end user.[18] In the absence of disinfection or some other selective conditions (eg, acidity), NTM are poor competitors for nutrients and are rarely found in natural waters.

Persistence of NTM in a flowing drinking water distribution or plumbing in homes, apartments, condominiums, hospitals, and buildings is owing to their surface hydrophobicity driving their attachment to pipe surfaces.[6] Although rich laboratory media are used for the cultivation of NTM in the laboratory, they are able to grow at low organic matter concentrations, namely, at 50 μg assimilable organic carbon per liter.[19] NTM growth in biofilms further increases their resistance to disinfection.[20] Piped water distribution systems are source of NTM in buildings.[18] Homes with a well water source (ie, groundwater) are found to have NTM less frequently.[21] Such infrequency of NTM in groundwaters likely reflects the filtration of water and the entrapment of particles and associated NTM in the smaller spaces and pores.

Proven sources of NTM, in which DNA fingerprints of patient and environmental NTM have been shown to be identical, include drinking water,[22] shower water,[1] and potting soil dusts.[2] Humans are likely to be exposed to NTM in their homes through the generation of aerosols in showers, water taps, hot tubs (spas), and humidifiers (both free standing and those part of a heating, ventilation, and air conditioning system). NTM are readily aerosolized because of their hydrophobic surface.[5] Dusts generated during potting plants or gardening are also likely sources of NTM infection.[2] This is particularly the case with dry potting soil, a product rich in NTM (1 million per gram).[2] In addition to household sources, water aerosols can be encountered at work, gyms, public places (fountains), cooling towers on buildings, and by rivers and streams (waterfalls). It is unlikely that NTM exposure can occur at the ocean shore because NTM numbers are quite low in ocean water (≥3% NaCl).[23]

Recently, the distribution of NTM disease cases across the United States was characterized and a number of "hot spots" of disease were identified.[24] Because the frequency of NTM disease was normalized by patient age, the areas with a high frequency of NTM disease did not reflect differences in population age groups.[24] Rather, this author would propose, the differences in NTM disease frequency reflect variation in the chemistry and microbiology of distribution systems and their water. Hot spots were identified in areas of the country rich in NTM whether natural, such as Louisiana and Florida acid, brown water swamps,[13] or human-engineered as in apartment/condominium-rich New York City.[25] Other "hot spots" included areas in which NTM surveys of water distribution systems have not been performed, such as the counties surrounding Santa Barbara, California. Areas of significantly lower NTM disease prevalence were found in the Desert Southwest and the Northern Great Plains. We can only speculate as to the basis for low NTM disease prevalence in those areas in the absence of NTM surveys of drinking water and drinking water quality—perhaps alkaline soils and hard water?

WHY DO NONTUBERCULOUS MYCOBACTERIA INHABIT THE HUMAN ENVIRONMENT?

The physiologic characteristics of the NTM are major determinants of its habitat occupancy. The surface hydrophobicity of NTM, owing to the lipid-rich outer membrane,[4] drives the attachment of cells to surfaces in both natural and human-engineered environments.[6] Attached cells, no matter how slowly growing, will not be washed out of a flowing system (eg, river or pipe). Hydrophobicity also drives the enrichment of NTM in aerosols above bodies of water[5] and is responsible, in part, for NTM's resistance to disinfectants.[7]

Factors contributing to the presence and growth of NTM in drinking water distribution systems and plumbing in buildings and homes include:

1. Impermeability to hydrophilic compounds such as disinfectants,[4]
2. Growth at low organic carbon concentrations,[19] and
3. The ability of NTM to metabolize complex organic compounds that are not metabolized by other drinking water microorganisms.[26]

The lack of movement and utilization of water in households and buildings when occupants are absent does not necessarily result in reduction in NTM numbers. Although such stagnant water is of low oxygen concentration as a result of O_2-consumption by water-borne microorganisms, NTM can still grow. The growth rates of M avium and M intracellulare at 12% oxygen is the same as in air (21% oxygen). M avium and M intracellulare can even grow, albeit at half the rate as air, at 6% oxygen (Lewis and Falkinham, unpublished data, 2014). In households, NTM heat resistance is a major factor in promoting persistence; for example, 90% of M avium cells survive after 60 minutes of exposure to 125°C (50°C).[11] Their heat resistance relative to other drinking water microbes very likely contributes to the very high numbers of NTM (100,000 colony-forming units per milliliter of water) in apartment/condominium buildings[25] or hospitals[27] with recirculating hot water systems.

NTM numbers are very high (1 million/gram) in peat-rich[2,12] and coastal acid soils.[13] Factors associated with those high numbers are high zinc concentrations and humic/fulvic acid concentrations.[13] As noted, NTM growth is stimulated by the presence of humic and fulvic acids.[14] Because NTM can grow within protozoa[16] and amoebae,[17] phagocytosis via grazing on microbial biofilms by free-living protists does not lead to NTM disappearance, but rather to increased numbers.

TRANSMISSION OF NONTUBERCULOUS MYCOBACTERIA

Routes that have been proposed for NTM transmission include (1) aerosolization and inhalation, (2) swallowing and aspiration, and (3) introduction into wounds, either through injury or surgical intervention (or both). To prove the existence of a transmission route, it is insufficient to simply isolate an NTM species or subspecies from both a patient and some environmental compartment (water or soil). Rather, to prove that one of those sources or routes was involved in infection requires the use of highly discriminatory fingerprinting tools. Although pulsed field gel electrophoresis comparisons have been employed for successfully identifying sources in the past,[22] pulsed field gel electrophoresis is time consuming and laborious. In contrast, *rep*-polymerase chain reaction (PCR)[28] and mycobacterial interspersed repetitive units–variable number of tandem repeats (MIRU-VNTR)[29] are simpler and highly discriminatory. The *rep*-PCR method takes advantage of the presence of interspersed repetitive sequences in mycobacterial DNA, providing a series of different sized PCR amplicons.[28] Counting the number of tandem repeats (ie, VNTR) of the MIRU generated by PCR also provides a number that can be recorded in a central database for strain comparisons by distant laboratories.[29] A second advantage of MIRU-VNTR typing is that it is superior to *rep*-PCR; specifically, isolates with the same *rep*-PCR patterns have been shown to have different MIRU-VNTR band patterns.[29] Because MIRU-VNTR typing is just starting to be employed, it remains to be seen whether it can provide sufficient discriminatory power to distinguish isolates of every NTM species.

Proven routes of NTM infection include (1) matching pulsed field gel electrophoresis patterns of *M avium* isolates from AIDS patients and Charles River water and drinking water in Boston,[22] (2) matching *rep*-PCR patterns of *M avium* isolates from a patient and their showerhead,[1] (3) *M avium*–infected patients and isolates from their household plumbing,[21] (4) NTM-infected patients

with sinusitis and their household plumbing biofilms,[25] and (5) identical 16S rRNA sequences of NTM isolates from patients and their potting soils.[2] Because of the widespread presence of NTM in drinking water distribution systems[18] and households[21] across the United States, one is led to the conclusion that most likely humans are almost always exposed to NTM. Infection is owing to exposure in an individual of increased susceptibility (eg, older slender women, heterozygotes for cystic fibrosis mutations, or those with reduced immunity).

AVOIDING NONTUBERCULOUS MYCOBACTERIA

The driver for identifying measures to avoid NTM exposure and infection is the fact that a substantial number of patients become reinfected with NTM, even after successful antibiotic therapy.[30] This is a consequence of the patient's continuing and increased susceptibility to NTM disease. To identify exposure-reduction measures, the approach in the Falkinham laboratory has been to identify factors that are associated with an absence of NTM in premises plumbing. That, in turn, is based on the assumption that NTM should be in every drinking water sample. Measures to reduce NTM numbers are in the provenance of providers of drinking water and homeowners.

For utilities, because NTM numbers are associated with water turbidity,[18] reduction in the turbidity of drinking water will reduce NTM numbers. NTM are hydrophobic and rather than residing suspended in water, they are attached to particles, especially if the source for drinking water is from surface lakes and rivers. Because NTM numbers are lower in ground waters (ie, wells),[21] selection of a ground water source for a utility could reduce NTM numbers in the distribution system. Evidence showing the role of organic matter in regulating *M avium* numbers,[19] suggests that reduction in organic matter content (eg, assimilable organic carbon) would be expected to reduce NTM numbers. In a pilot distribution system, it was shown that *M avium* failed to grow at assimilable organic carbon concentrations of less than 50 μg/L,[19] suggesting that organic matter reduction might serve to reduce NTM numbers. Whether that level of reduction of organic matter can be reached and if reached that measure will reduce NTM numbers awaits testing.

For homeowners and managers of large apartment/condominium buildings, **Box 2** lists measures that can be taken that may reduce NTM numbers. The suggestions are based on studies of factors influencing NTM numbers and trials have been initiated to test each. First, filtration at a tap or showerhead can prevent NTM passage. However, it is important to point out that not all "filters" prevent the passage of NTM. Specifically, granular-activated charcoal filters do not prevent the passage of NTM; their pores are too large.[31] Although effective in removing chlorine, metals, and organic compounds that can impart bad tastes to water, granular-activated charcoal filters can serve as an incubator of NTM, leading to the filter becoming a source of NTM.[31] Filters with pores small enough to prevent NTM passage are available, but they are expensive and require frequent replacement (30–60 days).

Recent research suggests 3 novel approaches that might be effective in reducing NTM numbers. First, household plumbing seldom had NTM if hot water heaters were set at 55°C (130°F) or higher.[21] The frequency of household water samples with NTM was significantly higher if the hot water heater was set at 50°C (125°F) or lower.[18] As of the date of this writing, only 1 trial of NTM reduction by increasing the temperature of a water heater has been attempted. In that trial, *M avium* disappeared from plumbing samples from a house after raising the hot water heater temperature. However, that was 1 trial and any recommendation must wait for further trials from parts of the United States whose water compositions differ.

Second, based on the observation that NTM numbers are low in water samples of high oxygen content,[13] a second possible approach to reduce NTM numbers would be to increase the oxygen content of premises plumbing. Because the actual break point for reduced NTM numbers was 2 mg/L and higher values can be attained through aeration of water without endangering occupants with bursting pipes, this approach will be tested in closed pilot systems.

Finally, in a study of showerheads across the United States, it was shown that the presence of pink-pigmented *Methylobacterium* was associated with the absence of *Mycobacterium*.[32] That finding was confirmed in a study of NTM patient households in Philadelphia (Falkinham, in preparation). Further, we have discovered that biofilms of methylobacteria inhibit the adherence of *M avium* to stainless steel (Falkinham, in preparation). The presence of pink slime in showers, shower curtains, and sinks is marker for the presence of *Methylobacterium* and a strong predictor of the absence of NTM. Although it is premature to suggest wholesale addition of methylobacteria to drinking water, the methylobacteria are normal, disinfectant-resistant inhabitants of drinking water. Further, because it seems that either methylobacteria or NTM are present in a plumbing sample—never together—a homeowner can usually find a tap or showerhead that has pink slime.

SUMMARY

NTM are opportunistic pathogens whose sources include drinking water, natural water, soils, and dusts. The NTM are not contaminants, but rather normal inhabitants of those habitats. Human infection occurs because NTM are in the same habitats that humans occupy and humans are thereby exposed to NTM in waters, aerosols, or dusts that can be inhaled or swallowed. Human-engineered habitats, such as a drinking water distribution system and premises plumbing select for and are ideal habitats for NTM. The NTM are much more resistant to common water disinfectants, such as chlorine, than are other microorganisms in drinking water. The use of disinfects thereby selects NTM persistence in drinking water distribution systems and household plumbing. In the absence of competitors that are killed by chlorine, NTM are free to exclusively use any nutrients for their growth. NTM patients are subject to reinfection, even after successful antibiotic therapy, owing to the fact that many, if not all, have a predisposing condition for NTM infection. Therefore, it is of value for water providers and homeowners to consider measures to reduce exposure to

NTM. Study of conditions affecting NTM presence or absence has identified several, including high hot water heater temperature that might reduce NTM numbers in drinking water and thereby exposure and infection.

REFERENCES

1. Falkinham JO III, Iseman MD, de Haas P, et al. *Mycobacterium avium* in a shower linked to pulmonary disease. J Water Health 2008;6:209–13.
2. De Groote MA, Pace NR, Fulton K, et al. Relationship between Mycobacterium isolates from patients with pulmonary mycobacterial infection and potting soils. Appl Environ Microbiol 2006;72:7602–6.
3. Tortoli E. Impact of genotypic studies on mycobacterial taxonomy: the new mycobacteria of the 1990s. Clin Microbiol Rev 2003;16:319–54.
4. Brennan PJ, Nikaido H. The envelope of mycobacteria. Annu Rev Biochem 1995;64:29–63.
5. Parker BC, Ford MA, Gruft H, et al. Epidemiology of infection by nontuberculous mycobacteria. IV. Preferential aerosolization of *Mycobacterium intracellulare* from natural waters. Am Rev Respir Dis 1983;128:652–6.
6. Mullis SN, Falkinham JO III. Adherence and biofilm formation of *Mycobacterium avium*, *Mycobacterium intracellulare* and Mycobacterium abscessus to household plumbing materials. J Appl Microbiol 2013;115:908–14.
7. Taylor RH, Falkinham JO III, Norton CD, et al. Chlorine-, chloramine-, chlorine dioxide- and ozone-susceptibility of *Mycobacterium avium*. Appl Environ Microbiol 2000;66:1702–5.
8. Rastogi N, Frehel C, Ryter A, et al. Multiple drug resistance in *Mycobacterium avium*: is the wall architecture responsible for the exclusion of antimicrobial agents? Antimicrob Agents Chemother 1981;20:666–77.
9. Bodner T, Miltner E, Bermudez LE. *Mycobacterium avium* resists exposure to the acidic conditions of the stomach. FEMS Microbiol Lett 2000;182:45–9.
10. Portaels F, Pattyn SR. Growth of mycobacteria in relation to the pH of the medium. Ann Microbiol (Paris) 1982;133:213–21.
11. Schulze-Röbbecke R, Buchholtz K. Heat susceptibility of aquatic mycobacteria. Appl Environ Microbiol 1992;58:1869–73.
12. Iivanainen EK, Martikainen PJ, Raisanen ML, et al. Mycobacteria in boreal coniferous forest soils. FEMS Microbiol Ecol 1997;23:325–32.
13. Kirschner RA Jr, Parker BC, Falkinham JO III. Epidemiology of infection by nontuberculous mycobacteria. X. *Mycobacterium avium*, *M. intracellulare*, and *M. scrofulaceum* in acid, brown-water swamps of the southeastern United States and their association with environmental variables. Am Rev Respir Dis 1992;145:271–5.
14. Kirschner RA, Parker BC, Falkinham JO III. Humic and fulvic acids stimulate the growth of *Mycobacterium avium*. FEMS Microbiol Ecol 1999;30:327–32.
15. Iivanainen E, Sallantaus T, Katila MJ, et al. Mycobacteria in run-off- waters from natural and drained peatlands. J Environ Qual 1999;28:1226–34.
16. Strahl ED, Gillaspy GE, Falkinham JO III. Fluorescent acid fast microscopy for measuring phagocytosis of *Mycobacterium avium*, *Mycobacterium intracellulare*, and *Mycobacterium scrofulaceum* by *Tetrahymena pyriformis* and their intracellular growth. Appl Environ Microbiol 2001;67:4432–9.
17. Cirillo JD, Falkow S, Tompkins LS, et al. Interaction of *Mycobacterium avium* with environmental amoebae enhances virulence. Infect Immun 1997;65:3759–67.
18. Falkinham JO III, Norton CD, LeChevallier MW. Factors influencing numbers of *Mycobacterium avium*, *Mycobacterium intracellulare*, and other mycobacteria in drinking water distribution systems. Appl Environ Microbiol 2001;67:1225–31.
19. Norton CD, LeChevallier MW, Falkinham JO III. Survival of *Mycobacterium avium* in a model distribution system. Water Res 2004;38:1457–66.
20. Steed KA, Falkinham JO III. Effect of growth in biofilms on chlorine susceptibility of *Mycobacterium avium* and *Mycobacterium intracellulare*. Appl Environ Microbiol 2006;72:4007–100.
21. Falkinham JO III. Nontuberculous mycobacteria from household plumbing of patients with nontuberculous mycobacteria disease. Emerg Infect Dis 2011;17:419–24.
22. von Reyn CF, Maslow JN, Barber TW, et al. Persistent colonisation of potable water as a source of *Mycobacterium avium* infection in AIDS. Lancet 1994;343:1137–41.
23. George KL, Parker BC, Gruft H, et al. Epidemiology of infection by nontuberculous mycobacteria. II. Growth and survival in natural waters. Am Rev Respir Dis 1980;122:89–94.
24. Adjemian J, Olivier KN, Seitz AE, et al. Spatial clusters of nontuberculous mycobacterial lung disease in the United States. Am J Respir Crit Care Med 2012;186:553–8.
25. Tichenor WS, Thurlow J, McNulty S, et al. Nontuberculous mycobacteria in household plumbing as possible cause of chronic rhinosinusitis. Emerg Infect Dis 2012;18:1612–7.
26. Krulwich TA, Pelliccione NJ. Catabolic pathways of coryneforms, nocardias, and mycobacteria. Annu Rev Microbial 1979;33:95–111.
27. duMoulin GC, Stottmeier KD, Pelletier PA, et al. Concentration of *Mycobacterium avium* by hospital hot water systems. J Am Med Assoc 1988;260:1599–601.
28. Cangelosi GA, Freeman RJ, Lewis KN, et al. Evaluation of a high-throughput repetitive-sequence-based PCR system for DNA fingerprinting of Mycobacterium

tuberculosis and *Mycobacterium avium* complex strains. J Clin Microbiol 2004;42:2685–93.

29. Iakhiaeva E, McNulty S, Brown-Elliott BA, et al. MIRU-VNTR of *Mycobacterium intracellulare* and *Mycobacterium chimaera* for strain comparison with establishment of a PCR-based data base. J Clin Microbiol 2013;51: 409–16.

30. Wallace RJ Jr, Zhang Y, Brown-Elliott BA, et al. Repeat positive cultures in *Mycobacterium intracellulare* lung disease after macrolide therapy represent new

infection in patients with bronchiectasis. J Infect Dis 2002;186:266–73.

31. Rodgers MR, Blackstone BJ, Reyes AL, et al. Colonisation of point of use water filters by silver resistant non-tuberculous mycobacteria. J Clin Pathol 1999; 52:629–32.

32. Feazel LM, Baumgartner LK, Peterson KL, et al. Opportunistic pathogens enriched in showerhead biofilms. Proc Natl Acad Sci U S A 2009;106: 16393–9.

Microbiological Diagnosis of Nontuberculous Mycobacterial Pulmonary Disease

Jakko van Ingen, MD, PhD

KEYWORDS

- Nontuberculous mycobacteria • Pulmonary disease • Microbiology • Diagnosis

KEY POINTS

- Despite its central role in the diagnosis of nontuberculous mycobacterial pulmonary disease, few studies have been performed to specifically address the optimization of microbiological diagnosis.
- Given their widespread environmental presence, isolation of nontuberculous mycobacteria (NTM) from specimens of nonsterile body sites such as the respiratory tract does not indicate disease per se.
- Diagnosis of NTM lung disease starts with procuring a good-quality respiratory sample.
- Both liquid and solid media should be incubated to increase sensitivity of culture.
- Clinical relevance differs by species; molecular identification of NTM isolates can aid in the distinction between occasional presence of NTM and true NTM lung disease.

BACKGROUND

Nontuberculous mycobacteria (NTM) are increasingly recognized as causative agents of mostly opportunistic infections of humans. Of all NTM diseases, pulmonary disease is by far the most frequent.[1] Other relatively common NTM diseases are skin infections after inoculation, cervical lymphadenitis in children, and disseminated disease in the severely immunocompromised.[1] Three distinct pulmonary disease manifestations are known: fibrocavitary disease, nodular bronchiectatic disease, and hypersensitivity pneumonitis. All 3 affect distinct patient categories.[2]

Given their widespread environmental presence, isolation of NTM from specimens of nonsterile body sites such as the respiratory tract does not indicate disease per se. Current diagnostic criteria presented in a Statement by the American Thoracic Society and Infectious Disease Society of America (ATS/IDSA) account for this discrepancy between isolation and disease. In short, to diagnose NTM pulmonary disease (NTM-PD), patients should have symptoms and radiologic signs suggestive of NTM-PD, and cultures of multiple respiratory tract samples must grow the same NTM species.[2]

Thus, clinicians and microbiologists face the task of acquiring optimal samples from the respiratory tract and making sure that NTM present in the sample are detected and identified. But what are the optimal methods to acquire and process the samples? And what could be the role of serology in diagnosing NTM-PD? This review summarizes currently available data on techniques involved in the microbiological diagnosis of NTM-PD, and aims to provide a framework for such optimal microbiological diagnosis.

Disclosure: None.
Department of Medical Microbiology (777), Radboud University Medical Center, PO Box 9101, 6500 HB Nijmegen, The Netherlands
E-mail addresses: jakko.vaningen@radboudumc.nl; vaningen.jakko@gmail.com

Clin Chest Med 36 (2015) 43–54
http://dx.doi.org/10.1016/j.ccm.2014.11.005
0272-5231/15/$ – see front matter © 2015 Elsevier Inc. All rights reserved.

LITERATURE REVIEW

The literature search was performed using the PubMed database (US National Library of Medicine; National Center for Biotechnology Information: http://www.ncbi.nlm.nih.gov/pubmed). The following Medical Subject Heading (MeSH) terms were used in the search, both alone and in combinations: "Mycobacterium/isolation and purification," "Mycobacterium/microbiology," "Mycobacterium avium-intracellulare Infection/diagnosis," "Mycobacterium Infections, Nontuberculous/diagnosis," and "Mycobacterium Infections, Nontuberculous/microbiology." Only English-language studies involving humans and published after 1990 were included. Case reports, case series, editorials, and literature reviews were excluded from analysis; the review focused on laboratory diagnostic studies. Reference lists of selected articles were searched for further articles for review.

SPECIMEN SUBMISSION

Given the central role of culture in the diagnosis of NTM lung disease, good diagnostics start with procuring a good-quality respiratory sample. Instruction of patients has been shown to increase the yield of acid-fast bacilli (AFB) smears for tuberculosis (TB) diagnostics; in a randomized study, well-instructed patients produced sputum samples of which 39% proved AFB-positive on direct microscopy, versus only 27% in the group that was not instructed.[3] Good instruction is therefore likely to be of benefit to NTM patients as well. The high prevalence of underlying chronic lung diseases in these patients[1,2] makes it likely that some patients have already been instructed on sputum expectoration. Hence, the added benefit may be smaller in NTM than in TB patients.

Visual inspection of the sputum sample is a helpful first assessment of its suitability. Saliva cultures are not useful to diagnose NTM-PD because NTM are occasionally present in the human oral cavity, where they may even be part of the normal commensal flora.[4] Thus, if a sample does not appear mucoid or purulent, it is best to request a new sample. Moreover, the purulence of a sputum sample may serve as a marker for disease severity, as it does in patients with bronchiectasis.[5]

The effect of delay in processing of sputum samples on the microscopy and culture results has not been investigated for NTM. *Mycobacterium tuberculosis* viability decreases if sputum samples are stored at room temperature. In one study, 163 sputum specimens of TB patients were split for immediate processing and storage for 3, 5, or 7 days. Smear microscopy results were not affected by storage duration, but although 92% of samples were culture-positive before storage, this rate diminished to 83% after 3 days of storage at room temperature.[6] In another study in 43 TB patients in Malawi, sputum storage at room temperature and at 4°C were compared; viability of cultures was best preserved by refrigeration, and significant losses in viability only appeared after more than 2 weeks of refrigeration.[7] Similar studies with sputum samples containing *Pseudomonas aeruginosa* showed that bacterial loads remained stable during storage at 4°C, decreased at −20°C, and increased during storage at 25°C for 48 hours.[8] Hence, samples are preferably incubated on relevant media on the same day.[2] Mailing samples to the laboratory is possible without significant losses in sputum yield if the time in the mail system is short (ie, <72 hours) and the sample arrives during normal laboratory opening hours.[9] If the latter fails, refrigeration on arrival is warranted.

HOW MANY SAMPLES AND AT WHICH INTERVALS?

For pulmonary TB diagnosis, the World Health Organization has long used the spot-morning-spot algorithm to obtain 3 consecutive sputum samples within a 24-hour period. After systematic reviews revealed that the increase in sensitivity brought about by the third sample was only 2%, only 2 sputum samples are now requested.[10] For the diagnosis of NTM-PD, this may not be very helpful. Temporary presence of an NTM species in the airways after environmental exposure may lead to consecutive positive samples, yet have no clinical significance. For this reason, the current ATS Statement on NTM disease states that "to establish the diagnosis of NTM lung disease, the collection of three early-morning specimens on different days is preferred."[2] Given the slow course of the disease, an interval of a week ensures that repeat positive cultures are unlikely to reflect a transient contamination of the airways after a single environmental exposure.

The rationale for the multiple sputum specimens and the prerequisite of having at least 2 positive cultures with the same species come largely from a study in Japan, which showed that radiologic evidence of disease (infiltrates or cavitary lesions) and progression was found in 98% of the patients who had 2 or more positive sputum cultures for *Mycobacterium avium* complex (MAC), versus just 2% in those with a single positive culture during 12 months of observation.[11] For 97% of patients, the first 2 positive cultures grew from the initial 3 sputum specimens. This approach may be less applicable to the nodular bronchiectatic type of NTM lung disease, as these patients tend to produce less or no sputum, and bacterial loads in sputum are generally lower.[2]

SPUTUM OR BRONCHOALVEOLAR LAVAGE?

Fibrocavitary NTM-PD is usually characterized by high bacterial burden, and sputum samples often suffice for the diagnosis.[2] Bronchoalveolar lavage (BAL) culture may be more sensitive than sputum culture in diagnosing nodular bronchiectatic NTM lung disease.[12] In a small study of 26 patients with suspected MAC nodular bronchiectatic lung disease, BAL yielded positive cultures in 13, compared with only 6 by sputum cultures.[13] In this specific circumstance a single positive culture from BAL, preferably with histologic evidence of mycobacterial disease, may be used to diagnose NTM lung disease. This approach is incorporated in the most recent statement by ATS/IDSA.[2] It must be emphasized that a diagnosis of NTM lung disease from a single positive BAL culture is only appropriate in patients who cannot produce adequate respiratory samples or whose sputum specimens do not grow mycobacteria. In addition, this only applies to NTM species strongly associated with human infections[2]; a single BAL culture of a rare or usually avirulent species should prompt an effort to obtain additional clinical samples.

MICROSCOPY

Three staining methods are commonly used to detect mycobacteria in respiratory samples: the auramine fluorochrome stain, and the carbol fuchsin-based Ziehl-Neelsen (ZN) and Kinyoun ("cold ZN") stains. NTM are as likely as M tuberculosis to be detected by fluorochrome staining.[14] The sensitivity of fluorochrome staining is generally higher than that of the carbol fuchsin staining procedures, but its specificity may be lower. Among the latter, ZN stains are more sensitive than Kinyoun stains, although these data are derived from M tuberculosis.[15] The sensitivity of these methods specifically for the diagnosis of NTM-PD has not been determined.

If direct microscopy reveals the presence of many squamous epithelial cells, the sample represents the oropharynx rather than the lower airways. The validity of such samples may be questioned, and can result in both false-positive and false-negative results. Ciliated epithelial cells or the presence of macrophages in a sample are signs that the sample comes from the lower respiratory tract.

DECONTAMINATION

Different protocols for decontamination of respiratory samples have been attempted. Decontamination by 1% N-acetyl-L-cysteine (NaLC)-NaOH is most commonly used. An increase in NaLC-NaOH concentrations from 1% to 1.25% lowers contamination rates but also leads to a 10% decrease in detection of mycobacteria in culture, and is not recommended.[16] Sulfuric acid (final concentration 3%) was recently shown to specifically improve detection rates of NTM, compared with 1% NaLC-NaOH, by liquid culture; this method did not improve the M tuberculosis detection rate.[17]

Samples from patients with cystic fibrosis (CF) differ in their chemical composition and their commensal flora, and may require different decontamination procedures to maximize their yield. In sputum samples from CF patients, decontamination by 0.25%/1% NaLC-NaOH, followed by 5% oxalic acid treatment, reduced the contamination rate from 74% of Lowenstein-Jensen slants or 36% of BacTec vials (for NaLC-NaOH alone) to only 5% and 3%[18]; however, in a multisite reproducibility study, this method performed well only in positive AFB smear samples.[19] Based on these findings, a prospective study compared NaLC-NaOH with NALC-NaOH followed by 5% oxalic acid treatment; although NaLC-NaOH with oxalic acid indeed reduced the contamination rate, it did not increase the yield of mycobacteria.[20] Subsequently, a second study of 920 samples from CF patients only applied NaLC-NaOH with oxalic acid in samples that yielded contaminated cultures after NALC-NaOH decontamination. This algorithm reduced contamination rates from 45% to 7% and did yield 10 additional positive cultures, in addition to 31 positive cultures obtained with NaLC-NaOH decontamination alone.[21] In a study comparing 1% chlorhexidine alone with 0.25%/1% NaLC-NaOH followed by 5% oxalic acid in 827 sputum samples from CF patients, the former yielded twice as many NTM-positive cultures (6.50% vs 3.25%), despite a higher contamination rate after chlorhexidine treatment (20% vs 14.2%); this study was only able to use solid Lowenstein-Jensen media for culture, as chlorhexidine has to be neutralized by lecithin to prevent inhibition of growth in liquid media. The lecithin generates nonspecific fluorescence in the Middlebrook 7H9 medium used in the Mycobacterium Growth Indicator Tube (MGIT) automated liquid culture system (BD Bioscience, Sparks, MD, USA), which is among the most commonly used liquid culture systems. The Lowenstein-Jensen medium is egg-based and thus contains egg lecithin.[22] The findings of the chlorhexidine method have now been independently confirmed. Nonetheless, in this second study the increased sensitivity of solid cultures after chlorhexidine decontamination was fully compensated for if NaLC-NaOH decontamination was performed and liquid cultures were incubated.[23]

MOLECULAR DETECTION OF NONTUBERCULOUS MYCOBACTERIA DIRECTLY IN RESPIRATORY SAMPLES

Molecular detection of NTM in respiratory samples is not common practice, especially in samples that are auramine-negative or ZN stain–negative. Several in-house assays have been developed and validated. The best described is a *Mycobacterium* genus–specific assay, used in conjunction with the COBAS Amplicor MTB assay (Roche Diagnostics, Rotkreuz, Switzerland), to discern *M tuberculosis* complex from NTM. This assay was tested in a study of 2169 samples, of which 77 were *M tuberculosis* complex–negative but *Mycobacterium* genus–positive, suggestive of NTM. By sequence analysis, 47 of these 77 (61%) proved to be NTM. Considering smear status and all culture results of the patient who submitted the sample, only 35 of the 77 *Mycobacterium* genus–positive samples (45%) were regarded as true positives. Eleven false-positive results were caused by *Corynebacterium* and *Gordonia* species.[24]

A commercial assay is now also available. The GenoType Mycobacteria Direct (GTMD; Hain Lifescience, Nehren, Germany) is a line probe assay that includes probes to detect the *M tuberculosis* complex but also *M avium*, *Mycobacterium intracellulare*, *Mycobacterium kansasii* and *Mycobacterium malmoense*. In early validation studies, mixed results were found. In one study using stored frozen ZN stain–positive sputum samples, 8 of 54 ZN-positive samples yielded *M avium* or *M kansasii* in culture that was not detected by the probe assay. Conversely, the GTMD identified *M intracellulare* in one sample that remained culture negative.[25] More recently, larger studies of fresh samples in areas of high TB endemicity have yielded largely similar results, showing limited (50%–60%) sensitivity of the GTMD assay in comparison with culture for detectable NTM species.[26,27]

CULTURE

Culture is still the mainstay of NTM-PD diagnosis. Thus, laboratories serving populations for whom NTM-PD is a health concern should optimize their mycobacterial culture methods to maximize the sensitivity of culture. This approach may demand investments to go beyond the methodologies used for tuberculosis diagnostics.

The selection of media, use of supplements, and incubation temperatures all affect the performance of culture, and are discussed in the following paragraphs.

Liquid Media, Solid Media, or Both?

For this analysis, the author has collected studies that have compared the performance of MGIT semiautomated liquid cultures with MGIT combined with 1 or more solid media. Comparative studies of other liquid media systems with solid media exist, but have studied systems that are no longer available (radiometric BacTec460 [BD Bioscience]) or systems that have since been technically upgraded (BacTalert [BioMerieux], VersaTrek [Trek Diagnostics]). The MGIT system is the most commonly used, certainly in Europe.

A total of 19 studies have examined the comparative performance of liquid culture alone versus liquid and solid culture. All studies were primarily interested in the performance for TB diagnostics, but do report their findings in NTM isolation. Ten of these studies had previously been incorporated in a meta-analysis.[28] From these studies, summarized in **Table 1**, it is evident that the use of a liquid and a solid medium, both incubated at 36° to 37°C, increases the sensitivity of NTM detection by culture by an average of 15% (range 0%–42%).[28–37]

Whereas the benefit of incubating a liquid and a solid medium is evident from the literature, the choice of solid medium is less evident. Most studies have only used Löwenstein-Jensen medium. In the few that applied multiple solid media and reported results per medium, the Löwenstein-Jensen medium was found to be most sensitive for the detection of NTM, superior to Middlebrook 7H10.[30,35]

An inherent limitation of automated liquid culture systems that has been studied in particular for the MGIT is the failure to detect slowly growing microorganisms with very low metabolic activity; this pertains particularly to some NTM species, most notably *Mycobacterium xenopi*. For laboratory practice, this implies that any culture flagged as negative has to be visually inspected before it is discarded, as subtle growth may have occurred. If growth is observed on inspection, molecular identification and a subculture must be performed.[38]

Supplemented Media: When and Which?

Two NTM species are notorious for their fastidiousness and requirement of supplemented media

Table 1
Sensitivity of culture algorithms using liquid media or liquid and solid media for NTM culture

Authors,[Ref.] Year	No. of Samples/ Patients	No. of NTM Isolates	Sensitivity MGIT (%)	Sensitivity MGIT + Solid Media (%)	Added Benefit (%)
Cruciani et al,[28] 2004[a]	14745	571	66	76	10
Chew et al,[29] 1998[a]	603/—	48 (only MAC)	94	98	4
Idigoras et al,[30] 2000[b]	2832/—	120	83	94	11
Sorlozano et al,[31] 2009[a]	1770/696	21	71	100	29
Rivera et al,[32] 1997[a]	202/100	12	58	100	42
Alcaide et al,[33] 2000[a]	1068/—	24	63	75	12
Lu et al,[34] 2002[a]	6062/—	213	88	100	12
Lee et al,[35] 2003[c]	1396/622	19	100	100	0
Sharp et al,[36] 2000[a]	2271/—	293	68	100	32
Hillemann et al,[37] 2006[d]	9558/—	259	86	100	14

Abbreviations: MAC, Mycobacterium avium complex; MGIT, Mycobacterium Growth Indicator Tube.
[a] Only Löwenstein-Jensen as solid medium.
[b] Löwenstein-Jensen, Coletsos, and Middlebrook 7H11 as solid media.
[c] Löwenstein-Jensen and Middlebrook 7H11 as solid media.
[d] Löwenstein-Jensen and Stonebrink as solid media.

to obtain growth: *Mycobacterium genavense* and *Mycobacterium haemophilum*.[39,40]

M genavense is very rarely a causative agent of NTM-PD. Its most frequent disease manifestation is a disseminated disease in the immunocompromised.[41] Cultivation of *M genavense* is possible in unsupplemented Middlebrook 7H9/MGIT medium, but cultures may need 12 weeks to grow and sensitivity is low. One option to improve its sensitivity is to lower the pH of the Middlebrook 7H9 medium to 5.5 or 6.0, for example using phosphoric acid.[42] In the only comparative study performed, 2 of 6 strains grew at pH 6.8, whereas all 6 grew at pH 6.0 and 5.5; the medium commercially available for pyrazinamide susceptibility testing of *M tuberculosis* also has a pH of 6.0 and is a good alternative.[42] Other groups have tried to optimize the Middlebrook 7H11 solid medium for cultivation of *M genavense*. Some success has been reported for supplementation of Middlebrook 7H11 with Mycobactin J.[43] For veterinary isolates, Realini and colleagues[39] have decreased the pH of the Middlebrook 7H11 medium to 6.2 and added yeast extract, sheep blood, and charcoal; this proved to be the most sensitive method for cultivation of their strains.

M haemophilum is also rarely a causative agent of NTM-PD.[44] The most frequent disease manifestations are disseminated disease with multiple nodular, ulcerative skin lesions in the severely immunocompromised,[40] and cervical lymphadenitis in immunocompetent children.[45] This species requires the addition of an iron source (hemin, ferric amonium citrate, factor X-V or other) to the medium for growth.

Incubation Temperature: 30°C, 37°C, or Both?

The optimal growth temperature differs for each NTM species. Most species have their growth optimum at 30°C; important exceptions for NTM-PD are *Mycobacterium abscessus*, which grows best at 37°C,[46] the MAC bacteria, which have a growth optimum at 36° to 42°C, and *M xenopi*, which has its growth optimum between 42° and 45°C.[47] Given the ambient temperature in the lower airways and lung tissue, it seems logical that NTM-PD in humans is predominantly caused by NTM that grow well at 37°C.

Few studies have examined the benefit of performing culture at different incubation temperatures. In the only prospective study, the BacTalert automated liquid culture system was used to incubate at both 30° and 37°C. Incubation at 30°C yielded faster growth, mainly of *Mycobacterium marinum*, and yielded one positive culture with *M marinum* that did not grow at 37°C. All *M marinum* isolates were cultured from skin biopsies.[48] The second study was a retrospective study of lymph node samples, whereby incubation at 30°C yielded more positive cultures for *M haemophilum* than incubation at 37°C.[45] Thus there seems to be no clear role for routine incubation of respiratory tract samples at 30°C, unless there is a specific suspicion of NTM-PD caused by a species that grows best at 30°C. This topic needs to be investigated in prospective studies.

Identification and the Evaluation of Clinical Relevance

The methods for identification of mycobacteria in clinical laboratories have changed dramatically over the past 2 decades. Currently applied methods and their relative cost are presented in **Table 2**.

Molecular methods have now surpassed biochemical tests and high-performance liquid chromatography of cell-wall mycolic acid content as methods of choice for NTM identification.[49] Two molecular methods are now commonly used. The first involves line probe assays, which are easy to perform, albeit costly, assays that allow a reasonable level of discrimination and will allow identification of the most frequently encountered species.[50] The second is (partial) gene sequencing, which allows a higher level of discrimination, often up to subspecies level, but is only feasible for laboratories with access to sequencing facilities. The target(s) selected for sequencing determine the discriminatory power: the *hsp65* and *rpoB* genes and the 16S-23S internal transcribed spacer (ITS) offer high discriminatory power and can identify up to subspecies level,[50–53] whereas 16S rRNA gene sequencing allows discrimination to species level for most species, or at least to complex level, particularly among the rapid growers (*Mycobacterium fortuitum* complex, *Mycobacterium chelonae–M abscessus* complex).[49,50]

Multilocus sequence-typing techniques have also been tested for NTM. Using this approach,

sequencing variable regions of several housekeeping genes has shown excellent identifications up to subspecies level (eg, for *M abscessus* subsp *abscessus* vs *M abscessus* subsp *bolletii* [formerly "*Mycobacterium bolletii*" and "*Mycobacterium massiliense*"]).[54,55] Apart from access to sequencing facilities, these methods are more difficult to implement because the analyses are more difficult and time-consuming and, thus, costly.

A new tool for species identification of NTM is matrix-assisted laser desorption ionization–time-of-flight (MALDI-TOF) mass spectrometry.[56] This technique is based on disruption of bacterial cells by laser and ionization of (mainly ribosomal) proteins, which are then pulled toward a detector. The time of flight of the various extracted proteins forms a spectrum of peaks that is species specific. Two commercial systems are now available and have had a tremendous impact in clinical bacteriology. Recently, procedures for lysis and protein extraction of mycobacteria have been standardized.[56] These procedures work well for pure cultures from strain collections. If applied to newly positive liquid cultures, only 50% of isolates can be immediately identified. For the remainder, subculture on solid media until the occurrence of visual growth is needed to obtain good MALDI-TOF results (J. van Ingen, unpublished data submitted for publication, 2014). The extraction protocols entail much hands-on work, which increases the cost of using this method. The discriminatory power of the MALDI-TOF method largely depends on the quality of its database, and this remains a drawback in comparison with the gene-sequencing methods whereby for most commonly used genetic targets, good (albeit not quality controlled) public databases are available.

Species identification is an indirect tool to assist in the diagnosis of NTM-PD, as NTM species differ in their clinical relevance.[1] In the Netherlands, this clinical relevance has been quantified, in retrospective studies, for all most commonly isolated NTM species. Clinical relevance was expressed as the percentage of patients with a positive culture from a respiratory sample yielding the NTM species under investigation, which ultimately met the ATS diagnostic criteria[2] and were thus considered to have definite NTM-PD. A visual representation of these findings is presented in **Fig. 1**. Isolation of *M kansasii* and (in northwestern Europe) *Mycobacterium szulgai* and *M malmoense* from pulmonary specimens indicates disease in more than 70% of all patients.[1,57,58] *Mycobacterium gordonae* and, to a lesser extent, *Mycobacterium simiae* or *M chelonae* are typically contaminants

Table 2
Identification methods for nontuberculous mycobacteria

Identification Assay	Discriminatory Power	Relative Cost
HPLC	+	$
Line probe assays	++	$$$$
16S rDNA gene sequencing	+++	$$$
Single-gene sequencing (other than 16S rDNA)	++++	$$$
Multigene sequencing	+++++	$$$$
MALDI-TOF	+++	$$

Abbreviations: HPLC, high-performance liquid chromatography; MALDI-TOF, matrix-assisted laser desorption ionization–time-of-flight mass spectrometry.

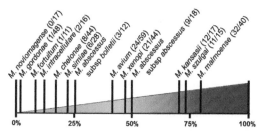

Fig. 1. Clinical relevance of nontuberculous mycobacteria isolated from respiratory samples in the Netherlands. (*Data from Refs.*[1,57–61])

rather than causative agents of true NTM-PD,[1,59,60] and MAC, *M xenopi*, and *M abscessus* form an intermediate category between these 2 extremes.[1,60,61] Similar studies on clinical relevance have been performed in other countries, where the results differ. In South Korea, *M kansasii* and *M szulgai* are isolated in frequencies similar to those reported in the Netherlands, but their clinical relevance is much lower.[62] Similarly, an early retrospective study in the United States addressed the clinical relevance of *M malmoense* isolation. This species was not only rarely isolated, it was also considered to be of clinical relevance in only 10% of the patients,[63] compared with in greater than 70% of patients in the Netherlands.[58]

Drug susceptibility testing of NTM is not covered in this review as it is not a diagnostic tool, although it may influence treatment decisions. Two recent reviews have covered this topic in detail.[64,65]

A "NEW KID ON THE BLOCK": SEROLOGY

In 2005, Seigo Kitada and colleagues[66] from Japan reported on the use of a serodiagnostic method for MAC-PD with an enzyme immunoassay (EIA) with MAC-specific glycopeptidolipid (GPL) core as the antigen. Significant increases in serum immunoglobulin (Ig)M, IgA, and IgG were measured in 106 patients with MAC-PD, compared with 11 with a single positive culture with MAC but no signs of disease, 30 patients with *M kansasii* PD, 77 patients with TB, and 126 healthy subjects. For anti-GPL IgA antibodies, sensitivity and specificity of 92.5% and 95.1% for diagnosing MAC-PD were measured, superior to those for IgG and IgM. The response levels also reflected the disease activity, as they decreased over time in patients who converted to negative cultures during treatment.[66] In a second study from the same group, anti-GPL core IgA antibody levels were measured in sera from 70 patients with MAC-PD, 18 with single MAC cultures in the absence of disease, 37 with pulmonary TB, 45 with other lung diseases, and 76 healthy controls. Setting the cutoff point for

the assay at 0.7 U/mL resulted in sensitivity and specificity for diagnosing MAC-PD of 84.3% and 100%, respectively. Significantly higher antibody levels were found in patients with nodular bronchiectatic disease than in patients with fibrocavitary disease.[67]

Follow-up studies by other groups showed slightly inferior results. Another group in Japan performed the assay in a cohort of 57 patients with MAC-PD, 18 patients with clinically suspected MAC-PD, 10 with single positive MAC cultures, 18 with pulmonary TB, 9 with other NTM disease, 18 with other lung diseases, and 20 healthy controls. The sensitivity and specificity of the assay to detect MAC-PD were 77% and 99%. The assay performed worse in immunocompromised patients. In addition, no correlations between the antibody level and disease type or radiologic extent of disease were found in patients with MAC-PD.[68] A subsequent study from South Korea demonstrated that the assay could not reliably distinguish MAC-PD from *M abscessus* PD, yet its sensitivity and specificity for discerning NTM-PD (MAC or *M abscessus*) from TB patients and healthy controls remained 77.5% and 100%.[69] A study from Taiwan reached the same conclusion from a cohort of 56 patients with MAC-PD, 11 with single positive MAC cultures, 13 with *M kansasii* PD, 26 with rapidly growing mycobacteria (RGM)-PD, 48 with pulmonary tuberculosis, and 42 household contacts of patients with TB. The overall sensitivity for detecting MAC-PD was 60%, with specificity of 87%; to distinguish MAC-PD from a single positive culture without clinical signs of MAC-PD the sensitivity was 60%, with specificity of 91%.[70] The only study outside East Asia was performed at National Jewish Health (Denver, CO, USA). There, in a cohort of 87 patients with definite MAC-PD (9 fibrocavitary, 78 nodular bronchiectatic), 13 with lung disease not caused by MAC, and 52 healthy volunteers, using a 0.3-U/mL cutoff, the sensitivity in detecting MAC-PD was 70%, with specificity of 94%. Using the 0.7-U/mL cutoff derived from previous studies, sensitivity and specificity only amounted to 52% and 94%. In this cohort, patients with *M intracellulare* PD had significantly higher IgA antibody titers than those with *M avium* PD.[71]

PERSPECTIVE

Despite its central role in NTM-PD diagnosis, few studies have been performed to specifically address the optimization of microbiological diagnosis. Even data on the most fundamental aspects, such as the impact of sample quality or time in transfer to the laboratory on sensitivity and specificity of microscopy and culture of sputum or BAL specimens for NTM-PD, have not been addressed in prospective studies. The lack of a gold standard for disease, other than meeting the ATS diagnostic criteria is, therefore, an important limitation.

The main message that emanates from the few available studies equates to George Fuechsel's informatics teaching mantra: "garbage in, garbage out."[72] Only timely submission of adequate volumes of (muco)purulent sputum samples obtained at least on separate days, but preferably days to a week apart, will enable the laboratory to perform good-quality culture and aid in applying the ATS diagnostic criteria. A practical algorithm is presented in **Fig. 2**.

For the laboratory, good-quality culture means that samples are preferably processed on the day of arrival, auramine and ZN staining is performed by trained microscopists, respiratory samples are decontaminated using the NaLC-NaOH method backed up by oxalic acid for heavily contaminated samples (eg, of CF patients), and at least a liquid and a solid culture medium are used. Based on currently available data, adding a solid medium to the frequently used MGIT automated liquid culture can lead to a gain in sensitivity of 15%, and is thus worthwhile. The addition of a solid medium does lead to an increase in the cost of diagnostics. This cost should be appreciated in the context of the total cost of diagnosis

and treatment of NTM-PD. The cost of treating NTM-PD on an outpatient basis amounted to a median of $499 per month of treatment, $321 for medication, and $144 for nonmedication cost, in Canada in 2008 (equal to €354 or US$459).[73] A study performed in the United States measured similar median monthly costs, at US$481.[74] The added benefit probably outweighs the cost of adding solid media.

Optimizing the microbiological diagnosis of NTM-PD may start with simple measures such as changing the laboratory forms, electronic or paper, to include a tick box to request culture specifically for nontuberculous mycobacteria along with one for *M tuberculosis* complex. In settings where NTM disease is as prevalent or more prevalent than TB, the reverse may be helpful; ticking the sole "mycobacterium culture" should prompt the laboratory to perform culture on liquid and solid media. Submission of skin or lymph node biopsies should prompt the laboratory to also set up cultures at lower (ie, 30°C) incubation temperatures.[48]

One of the complicating factors in diagnostics is that it demands clinicians to recognize NTM-PD and then request relevant diagnostics. NTM will not likely be detected in routine bacteriologic workup if no mycobacterial culture is requested. On the other hand, if a single sputum specimen is to be processed for routine bacterial culture, fungal culture, and mycobacterial culture, the volume of sputum available for each individual test

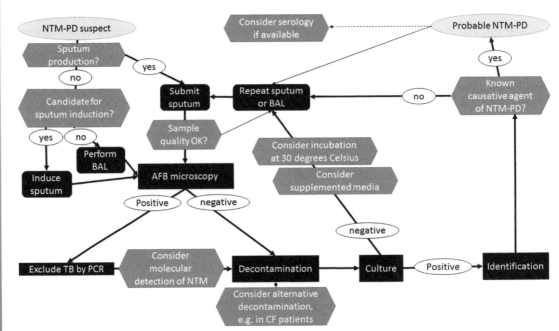

Fig. 2. Proposed algorithm for optimizing microbiological diagnosis of nontuberculous mycobacterial pulmonary disease (NTM-PD). AFB, acid-fast bacilli; BAL, bronchoalveolar lavage; CF, cystic fibrosis; PCR, polymerase chain reaction; TB, tuberculosis.

will be low, which likely has a negative impact on sensitivity.[75] This fundamental aspect of microbiological NTM-PD diagnosis also awaits study.

The potential role for serology deserves further study. The currently available assay seems to detect the most common manifestations of MAC-PD (nodular bronchiectatic and fibrocavitary disease) with reasonable sensitivity and specificity. However, it has been studied in few settings. It seems to perform best in nodular bronchiectatic diseases[66,67] and, in one study, better in *M intracellulare* than in *M avium* disease.[71] In many settings, *M avium* is the predominant MAC organism observed in clinical practice.[76] Moreover, in some settings the fibrocavitary *M avium* PD is most frequent.[1] The performance of this serodiagnostic assay needs to be evaluated in these various settings.

REFERENCES

1. van Ingen J, Bendien SA, de Lange WC, et al. Clinical relevance of nontuberculous mycobacteria isolated in the Nijmegen-Arnhem region, the Netherlands. Thorax 2009;64:502–6.

2. Griffith DE, Aksamit T, Brown-Elliot BA, et al. An official ATS/IDSA statement: diagnosis, treatment, and prevention of nontuberculous mycobacterial diseases. Am J Respir Crit Care Med 2007;175: 367–416.

3. Alisjahbana B, van Crevel R, Danusantoso H, et al. Better patient instruction for sputum sampling can improve microscopic tuberculosis diagnosis. Int J Tuberc Lung Dis 2005;9:814–7.

4. Wali SO, Abdelaziz MM, Krayem AB, et al. The presence of atypical mycobacteria in the mouthwashes of normal subjects: role of tap water and oral hygiene. Ann Thorac Med 2008;3:5–8.

5. Goeminne PC, Vandooren J, Moelants EA, et al. The sputum colour chart as a predictor of lung inflammation, proteolysis and damage in non-cystic fibrosis bronchiectasis: a case-control analysis. Respirology 2014;19:203–10.

6. Paramasivan CN, Narayana AS, Prabhakar R, et al. Effect of storage of sputum specimens at room temperature on smear and culture results. Tubercle 1983;64:119–24.

7. Banda HT, Harries AD, Boeree MJ, et al. Viability of stored sputum specimens for smear microscopy and culture. Int J Tuberc Lung Dis 2000;4:272–4.

8. Murray MP, Doherty CJ, Govan JR, et al. Do processing time and storage of sputum influence quantitative bacteriology in bronchiectasis? J Med Microbiol 2010;59:829–33.

9. Pye A, Hill SL, Bharadwa P, et al. Effect of storage and postage on recovery and quantitation of bacteria in sputum samples. J Clin Pathol 2008;61:352–4.

10. Mase SR, Ramsay A, Ng V, et al. Yield of serial sputum specimen examinations in the diagnosis of pulmonary tuberculosis: a systematic review. Int J Tuberc Lung Dis 2007;11:485–95.

11. Tsukamura M. Diagnosis of disease caused by *Mycobacterium avium* complex. Chest 1991;99: 667–9.

12. Sugihara E, Hirota N, Niizeki T, et al. Usefulness of bronchial lavage for the diagnosis of pulmonary disease caused by *Mycobacterium avium-intracellulare* complex (MAC) infection. J Infect Chemother 2003; 9:328–32.

13. Tanaka E, Amitani R, Niimi A, et al. Yield of computed tomography and bronchoscopy for the diagnosis of *Mycobacterium avium* complex pulmonary disease. Am J Respir Crit Care Med 1997;155: 2041–6.

14. Wright PW, Wallace RJ Jr, Wright NW, et al. Sensitivity of fluorochrome microscopy for detection of *Mycobacterium tuberculosis* versus nontuberculous mycobacteria. J Clin Microbiol 1998;36:1046–9.

15. Somoskövi A, Hotaling JE, Fitzgerald M, et al. Lessons from a proficiency testing event for acid-fast microscopy. Chest 2001;120:250–7.

16. Peres RL, Maciel EL, Morais CG, et al. Comparison of two concentrations of NALC-NaOH for decontamination of sputum for mycobacterial culture. Int J Tuberc Lung Dis 2009;13:1572–5.

17. Buijtels PC, Petit PL. Comparison of NaOH-N-acetyl cysteine and sulfuric acid decontamination methods for recovery of mycobacteria from clinical specimens. J Microbiol Methods 2005;62:83–8.

18. Whittier S, Hopfer RL, Knowles MR, et al. Improved recovery of mycobacteria from respiratory secretions of patients with cystic fibrosis. J Clin Microbiol 1993;31:861–4.

19. Whittier S, Olivier K, Gilligan P, et al. Proficiency testing of clinical microbiology laboratories using modified decontamination procedures for detection of nontuberculous mycobacteria in sputum samples from cystic fibrosis patients. J Clin Microbiol 1997; 35:2706–8.

20. Bange FC, Kirschner P, Böttger EC. Recovery of mycobacteria from patients with cystic fibrosis. J Clin Microbiol 1999;37:3761–3.

21. Bange FC, Bottger EC. Improved decontamination method for recovering mycobacteria from patients with cystic fibrosis. Eur J Clin Microbiol Infect Dis 2002;21:546–8.

22. Ferroni A, Vu-Thien H, Lanotte P, et al. Value of the chlorhexidine decontamination method for recovery of nontuberculous mycobacteria from sputum samples of patients with cystic fibrosis. J Clin Microbiol 2006;44:2237–9.

23. De Bel A, De Geyter D, De Schutter I, et al. Sampling and decontamination method for culture of nontuberculous mycobacteria in respiratory samples of

cystic fibrosis patients. J Clin Microbiol 2013;51: 4204–6.

24. Peter-Getzlaff S, Lüthy J, Voit A, et al. Detection and identification of *Mycobacterium* spp. in clinical specimens by combining the Roche Cobas Amplicor *Mycobacterium tuberculosis* assay with Mycobacterium genus detection and nucleic acid sequencing. J Clin Microbiol 2010;48(11):3943–8.

25. Seagar AL, Prendergast C, Emmanuel FX, et al. Evaluation of the genotype mycobacteria direct assay for the simultaneous detection of the *Mycobacterium tuberculosis* complex and four atypical mycobacterial species in smear-positive respiratory specimens. J Med Microbiol 2008;57:605–11.

26. Bicmen C, Gunduz AT, Coskun M, et al. Molecular detection and identification of *Mycobacterium tuberculosis* complex and four clinically important nontuberculous mycobacterial species in smear-negative clinical samples by the genotype mycobacteria direct test. J Clin Microbiol 2011;49:2874–8.

27. Luetkemeyer AF, Kendall MA, Wu X, et al, Adult AIDS Clinical Trials Group A5255 Study Team. Evaluation of two line probe assays for rapid detection of *Mycobacterium tuberculosis*, tuberculosis (TB) drug resistance, and non-TB mycobacteria in HIV-infected individuals with suspected TB. J Clin Microbiol 2014; 52:1052–9.

28. Cruciani M, Scarparo C, Malena M, et al. Meta-analysis of BACTEC MGIT 960 and BACTEC 460 TB, with or without solid media, for detection of mycobacteria. J Clin Microbiol 2004;42:2321–5.

29. Chew WK, Lasaitis RM, Schio FA, et al. Clinical evaluation of the Mycobacteria Growth Indicator Tube (MGIT) compared with radiometric (Bactec) and solid media for isolation of *Mycobacterium* species. J Med Microbiol 1998;47:821–7.

30. Idigoras P, Beristain X, Iturzaeta A, et al. Comparison of the automated nonradiometric Bactec MGIT 960 system with Löwenstein-Jensen, Coletsos, and Middlebrook 7H11 solid media for recovery of mycobacteria. Eur J Clin Microbiol Infect Dis 2000;19:350–4.

31. Sorlozano A, Soria I, Roman J, et al. Comparative evaluation of three culture methods for the isolation of mycobacteria from clinical samples. J Microbiol Biotechnol 2009;19:1259–64.

32. Rivera AB, Tupasi TE, Grimaldo ER, et al. Rapid and improved recovery rate of Mycobacterium tuberculosis in Mycobacteria Growth Indicator Tube combined with solid Löwenstein Jensen medium. Int J Tuberc Lung Dis 1997;1:454–9.

33. Alcaide F, Benítez MA, Escribà JM, et al. Evaluation of the BACTEC MGIT 960 and the MB/BacT systems for recovery of mycobacteria from clinical specimens and for species identification by DNA AccuProbe. J Clin Microbiol 2000;38:398–401.

34. Lu D, Heeren B, Dunne WM. Comparison of the automated mycobacteria growth indicator tube system (BACTEC 960/MGIT) with Löwenstein-Jensen medium for recovery of mycobacteria from clinical specimens. Am J Clin Pathol 2002;118:542–5.

35. Lee JJ, Suo J, Lin CB, et al. Comparative evaluation of the BACTEC MGIT 960 system with solid medium for isolation of mycobacteria. Int J Tuberc Lung Dis 2003;7:569–74.

36. Sharp SE, Lemes M, Sierra SG, et al. Löwenstein-Jensen media. No longer necessary for mycobacterial isolation. Am J Clin Pathol 2000;113:770–3.

37. Hillemann D, Richter E, Rüsch-Gerdes S. Use of the BACTEC Mycobacteria Growth Indicator Tube 960 automated system for recovery of mycobacteria from 9,558 extrapulmonary specimens, including urine samples. J Clin Microbiol 2006;44:4014–7.

38. Piersimoni C, Nista D, Bornigia S, et al. Unreliable detection of *Mycobacterium xenopi* by the nonradiometric Bactec MGIT 960 culture system. J Clin Microbiol 2009;47:804–6.

39. Realini L, de Ridder K, Hirschel B, et al. Blood and charcoal added to acidified agar media promote the growth of *Mycobacterium genavense*. Diagn Microbiol Infect Dis 1999;34:45–50.

40. Saubolle MA, Kiehn TE, White MH, et al. *Mycobacterium haemophilum*: microbiology and expanding clinical and geographic spectra of disease in humans. Clin Microbiol Rev 1996;9:435–47.

41. Hoefsloot W, van Ingen J, Peters EJ, et al. *Mycobacterium genavense* in the Netherlands: an opportunistic pathogen in HIV and non-HIV immunocompromised patients. An observational study in 14 cases. Clin Microbiol Infect 2013;19:432–7.

42. Thomsen VO, Dragsted UB, Bauer J, et al. Disseminated infection with *Mycobacterium genavense*: a challenge to physicians and mycobacteriologists. J Clin Microbiol 1999;37:3901–5.

43. Coyle MB, Carlson LC, Wallis CK, et al. Laboratory aspects of "*Mycobacterium genavense*", a proposed species isolated from AIDS patients. J Clin Microbiol 1992;30:3206–12.

44. Swart RM, van Ingen J, van Soolingen D, et al. Nontuberculous *Mycobacterium* infection and tumor necrosis factor-α antagonists. Emerg Infect Dis 2009;15:1700–1.

45. Bruijnesteijn van Coppenraet LE, Kuijper EJ, Lindeboom JA, et al. *Mycobacterium haemophilum* and lymphadenitis in children. Emerg Infect Dis 2005;11:62–8.

46. Moore M, Frerichs JB. An unusual acid-fast infection of the knee with subcutaneous, abscess-like lesions of the gluteal region; report of a case with a study of the organism, *Mycobacterium abscessus*, n. sp. J Invest Dermatol 1953;20:133–69.

47. Torkko P, Suomalainen S, Iivanainen E, et al. *Mycobacterium xenopi* and related organisms isolated from stream waters in Finland and description of *Mycobacterium botniense* sp. nov. Int J Syst Evol Microbiol 2000;50:283–9.

48. Alfa MJ, Manickam K, Sepehri S, et al. Evaluation of BacT/Alert 3D automated unit for detection of nontuberculous mycobacteria requiring incubation at 30 degrees C for optimal growth. J Clin Microbiol 2011;49:2691–3.

49. Springer B, Stockman L, Teschner K, et al. Two-laboratory collaborative study on identification of mycobacteria: molecular versus phenotypic methods. J Clin Microbiol 1996;34:296–303.

50. De Zwaan R, van Ingen J, van Soolingen D. Utility of rpoB gene sequencing for identification of nontuberculous mycobacteria in the Netherlands. J Clin Microbiol 2014;52:2544–51.

51. Roth A, Fischer M, Hamid ME, et al. Differentiation of phylogenetically related slowly growing mycobacteria based on 16S-23S rRNA gene internal transcribed spacer sequences. J Clin Microbiol 1998; 36:139–47.

52. McNabb A, Eisler D, Adie K, et al. Assessment of partial sequencing of the 65-kilodalton heat shock protein gene (hsp65) for routine identification of Mycobacterium species isolated from clinical sources. J Clin Microbiol 2004;42:3000–11.

53. Adékambi T, Colson P, Drancourt M. rpoB-based identification of nonpigmented and late-pigmenting rapidly growing mycobacteria. J Clin Microbiol 2003;41:5699–708.

54. Macheras E, Roux AL, Bastian S, et al. Multilocus sequence analysis and rpoB sequencing of Mycobacterium abscessus (sensu lato) strains. J Clin Microbiol 2011;49:491–9.

55. Zelazny AM, Root JM, Shea YR, et al. Cohort study of molecular identification and typing of Mycobacterium abscessus, Mycobacterium massiliense, and Mycobacterium bolletii. J Clin Microbiol 2009;47: 1985–95.

56. Buchan BW, Riebe KM, Timke M, et al. Comparison of MALDI-TOF MS with HPLC and nucleic acid sequencing for the identification of Mycobacterium species in cultures using solid medium and broth. Am J Clin Pathol 2014;141:25–34.

57. van Ingen J, Boeree MJ, de Lange WC, et al. Clinical relevance of Mycobacterium szulgai in the Netherlands. Clin Infect Dis 2008;46:1200–5.

58. Hoefsloot W, van Ingen J, de Lange WC, et al. Clinical relevance of Mycobacterium malmoense isolation in the Netherlands. Eur Respir J 2009;34:926–31.

59. van Ingen J, Boeree MJ, Dekhuijzen PN, et al. Clinical relevance of Mycobacterium simiae in pulmonary samples. Eur Respir J 2008;31:106–9.

60. van Ingen J, de Zwaan R, Dekhuijzen R, et al. Clinical relevance of Mycobacterium chelonae-abscessus group isolation in 95 patients. J Infect 2009;59: 324–31.

61. van Ingen J, Boeree MJ, de Lange WC, et al. Mycobacterium xenopi clinical relevance and determinants, the Netherlands. Emerg Infect Dis 2008;14:385–9.

62. Koh WJ, Kwon OJ, Jeon K, et al. Clinical significance of nontuberculous mycobacteria isolated from respiratory specimens in Korea. Chest 2006; 129:341–8.

63. Buchholz UT, McNeil MM, Keyes LE, et al. Mycobacterium malmoense infections in the United States, January 1993 through June 1995. Clin Infect Dis 1998;27:551–8.

64. van Ingen J, Boeree M, van Soolingen D, et al. Resistance mechanisms and drug susceptibility testing of nontuberculous mycobacteria. Drug Resist Updat 2012;15:149–61.

65. Brown-Elliott BA, Nash KA, Wallace RJ Jr. Antimicrobial susceptibility testing, drug resistance mechanisms, and therapy of infections with nontuberculous mycobacteria. Clin Microbiol Rev 2012;25:545–82.

66. Kitada S, Maekura R, Toyoshima N, et al. Use of glycopeptidolipid core antigen for serodiagnosis of Mycobacterium avium complex pulmonary disease in immunocompetent patients. Clin Diagn Lab Immunol 2005;12:44–51.

67. Kitada S, Kobayashi K, Ichiyama S, et al, MAC Serodiagnosis Study Group. Serodiagnosis of Mycobacterium avium-complex pulmonary disease using an enzyme immunoassay kit. Am J Respir Crit Care Med 2008;177:793–7.

68. Kobashi Y, Mouri K, Obase Y, et al. Serological assay by use of glycopeptidolipid core antigen for Mycobacterium avium complex. Scand J Infect Dis 2013;45:241–9.

69. Jeong BH, Kim SY, Jeon K, et al. Serodiagnosis of Mycobacterium avium complex and Mycobacterium abscessus complex pulmonary disease by use of IgA antibodies to glycopeptidolipid core antigen. J Clin Microbiol 2013;51:2747–9.

70. Shu CC, Ato M, Wang JT, et al. Sero-diagnosis of Mycobacterium avium complex lung disease using serum immunoglobulin A antibody against glycopeptidolipid antigen in Taiwan. PLoS One 2013;8: e80473.

71. Kitada S, Levin A, Hiserote M, et al. Serodiagnosis of Mycobacterium avium complex pulmonary disease in the USA. Eur Respir J 2013;42:454–60.

72. Butler J, Lidwell W, Holden K, editors. Universal principles of design. 2nd edition. Gloucester (MA): Rockport Publishers; 2010. p. 112. ISBN 1-59253-587-9.

73. Leber A, Marras TK. The cost of medical management of pulmonary nontuberculous mycobacterial disease in Ontario, Canada. Eur Respir J 2011;37: 1158–65.

74. Ballarino GJ, Olivier KN, Claypool RJ, et al. Pulmonary nontuberculous mycobacterial infections: antibiotic treatment and associated costs. Respir Med 2009;103:1448–55.

75. Fraczek MG, Kirwan MB, Moore CB, et al. Volume dependency for culture of fungi from respiratory

secretions and increased sensitivity of Aspergillus quantitative PCR. Mycoses 2014;57:69–78.

76. Hoefsloot W, van Ingen J, Andrejak C, et al, Nontuberculous Mycobacteria Network European Trials Group. The geographic diversity of nontuberculous mycobacteria isolated from pulmonary samples: an NTM-NET collaborative study. Eur Respir J 2013; 42:1604–13.

Medications and Monitoring in Nontuberculous Mycobacteria Infections

Eric F. Egelund, PharmD, PhD[a], Kevin P. Fennelly, MD, MPH[b], Charles A. Peloquin, PharmD[a],*

KEYWORDS

- Nontuberculous mycobacteria • *Mycobacterium avium* complex • Macrolides • Ethambutol
- Rifamycins • β-Lactams • Pharmacokinetics

KEY POINTS

- In general, multiple drugs are needed to treat nontuberculous mycobacteria (NTM) infections in order to prevent the selection of drug resistance.
- Pharmacokinetic and especially pharmacodynamic indices are not well established for NTM infections.
- Because of the lack of agents specifically developed for NTM, and the lack of pharmacodynamic indices for the currently available drugs, treatment is long and often ineffective.
- Prospective studies are needed to determine appropriate drug regimens for most NTM species.

INTRODUCTION

Nontuberculous mycobacteria (NTM) encompass more than 200 species of bacteria. Of these, only a small number of species are known to cause human disease; most commonly *Mycobacterium avium* complex (MAC), *Mycobacterium kansasii* and the *Mycobacterium abscessus* group. MAC and *M kansasii* are slow-growing mycobacteria. Doubling times for these mycobacteria approach 1 day, and they may take longer than a week to form mature colonies.[1] These infections often are treated with macrolides plus other antimycobacterial drugs, such as ethambutol, rifampin, or rifabutin. Another major group are the rapidly growing mycobacteria, which include *M abscessus* (including *M*

abscessus subsp. *bolletii* and *M abscessus* subsp. *abscessus*), *Mycobacterium chelonae*, and *Mycobacterium fortuitum*.[2] Drug regimens for the rapidly growing mycobacteria depart significantly from the treatment of *Mycobacterium tuberculosis* (Mtb) or MAC.

The drugs used for the treatment of these infections were not designed specifically for NTM. The rationale for their use has often been extrapolated from the treatment of tuberculosis. Many of the prospective studies for NTM were conducted in patients with acquired immunodeficiency syndrome (AIDS) with disseminated MAC, before the advent of highly active antiretroviral therapy. It is not known whether the study results from disseminated MAC infections in patients with AIDS can be

Disclosures: None.
[a] Infectious Disease Pharmacokinetics Laboratory, College of Pharmacy, and Emerging Pathogens Institute, University of Florida, 1600 Southwest Archer Road, Gainesville, FL 32610-0486, USA; [b] College of Medicine, and Emerging Pathogens Institute, University of Florida, 1600 Southwest Archer Road, Gainesville, FL 32610-0486, USA
* Corresponding author. Infectious Disease Pharmacokinetics Laboratory, College of Pharmacy, University of Florida, 1600 Southwest Archer Road, Room P4-33, PO Box 100486, Gainesville, FL 32610-0486.
E-mail address: peloquin@cop.ufl.edu

Clin Chest Med 36 (2015) 55–66
http://dx.doi.org/10.1016/j.ccm.2014.11.001
0272-5231/15/$ – see front matter © 2015 Elsevier Inc. All rights reserved.

extrapolated to other situations, such as nodular bronchiectatic lung infections in elderly women. Randomized clinical trials for pulmonary NTM are rare in such patients, or those with chronic obstructive pulmonary disease. Understanding of the treatment of pulmonary NTM infections is limited, and is based largely on trial and error: Treatment usually lasts months to years. Long-term monotherapy leads to drug resistance. Drug combinations are needed to prevent resistance.[3]

NTM infections are increasingly common in the elderly, and age-related changes in drug absorption, metabolism, and excretion may lead to decreased efficacy and increased toxicity.[4] The extended durations of treatment often lead to adverse drug reactions, drug interactions, and patient nonadherence or treatment discontinuation. Given these obstacles, it is imperative that clinicians begin to optimize the use of these drugs, and find better drugs.

This issue discusses specific treatment regimens for the slow-growing and rapidly growing mycobacteria, as well as treatment in special populations. This article provides information about the drugs commonly used to treat NTM, the use of therapeutic drug monitoring (TDM), and clinical monitoring for adverse drug reactions.

MACROLIDES

The macrolides (clarithromycin and azithromycin) are the cornerstones of treatment of most slow-growing NTM infections. Some rapidly growing NTM can be treated with macrolides, but *M fortuitum* and *M abscessus* often are macrolide resistant because of the presence of the *erm* gene.[5] Isolates from previously treated patients with NTM also show higher rates of macrolide resistance, making any subsequent treatment far less likely to succeed. Therefore, it is necessary to avoid macrolide monotherapy, and it is necessary to make the initial NTM treatment as effective as possible in order to prevent macrolide resistance.[6]

Macrolides bind to the 50S subunit of bacterial ribosomes and prevent protein synthesis. Typical clarithromycin minimal inhibitory concentrations (MICs) for MAC isolates are 1 to 4 μg/mL.[7] Clarithromycin has been more commonly used than azithromycin because it has been studied more extensively. However, clarithromycin is both a substrate for and inhibitor of cytochrome P (CYP) 3A enzymes, whereas azithromycin is not. Thus, azithromycin often is preferred in order to avoid drug interactions, including with the rifamycins.

Clarithromycin generally is dosed at 500 mg twice daily, producing peak concentrations (C_{max}) of 2 to 7 μg/mL 2 to 3 hours after the dose (time of peak [T_{max}]). Azithromycin is dosed at 250 mg or, more often, 500 mg daily, producing C_{max} of 0.2 to 0.7 μg/mL (10-fold lower than clarithromycin) and a T_{max} about 2 hours after the dose. Macrolide tissue concentrations are far greater than serum concentrations: 2-fold to 20-fold greater with clarithromycin and 10-fold to 100-fold greater for azithromycin.[8] As noted, clarithromycin is metabolized by CYP3A4. Its primary metabolite, 14-hydroxy-clarithromycin, is not active against most NTM. Therefore, unlike *Haemophilus influenzae* infections, the clarithromycin metabolite does not seem to contribute to treatment. Combinations with rifamycins, especially rifampin, convert much of clarithromycin to the 14-OH form, and this likely detracts from therapy.

Food has minor effects on absorption of clarithromycin, slightly delaying T_{max}, increasing C_{max} by 24%, and reducing its area under the concentration versus time curve (AUC) by only 11%.[9] Food has similarly minor effects on azithromycin oral tablet absorption, increasing C_{max} by 23% (or by 56% for the azithromycin oral suspension).[10] With either formulation, the azithromycin AUC remains largely unchanged. Note that the azithromycin extended-release oral suspension is not bioequivalent to the immediate-release formulation (83% relative bioavailability), and therefore cannot be used interchangeably.[10]

Gastrointestinal (GI) disturbances are the most common adverse effect seen with the macrolides. Diarrhea, nausea/vomiting, and abdominal pain often are reported.[11] Switching macrolides (from clarithromycin to azithromycin, or vice versa) may be tried, or antiemetics may be tried if that fails. Azithromycin and clarithromycin are both associated with QT prolongation.[12–14] In 2013, the US Food and Drug Administration (FDA) issued a warning regarding azithromycin use and the risk of fatal heart rhythms.[15,16] In 2014, a large observational study of Danish patients showed an increased risk of cardiac death in patients taking clarithromycin compared with those taking penicillin V.[17] Macrolide use should be used with caution in patients with underlying heart disease, electrolyte abnormalities, or those taking other medications that can prolong the QT interval.[18]

RIFAMYCINS (RIFAMPIN/RIFABUTIN)

The rifamycins have broad antimicrobial coverage and are often used in the treatment of NTM infections. Rifamycins inhibit DNA-dependent RNA-polymerase, which prevents transcription of DNA to RNA.[19] The rifamycins show concentration-dependent killing of mycobacteria. Therefore, increasing exposure increases efficacy and reduces resistance.[20] The current usual rifampin dose is 10 mg/kg. A rifampin oral dose of 600 mg yields a C_{max} of 8 to 24 μg/mL approximately 2 hours after the dose.[21] Food reduces the C_{max} approximately 35%, with little effect on the AUC. Thus, rifampin should be given on an empty stomach.[22] Reduced or delayed absorption may occur with certain disease states, particularly diabetes, human immunodeficiency virus (HIV), and cystic fibrosis.[23,24]

Treatment can be particularly difficult to manage in patients with HIV coinfected with MAC. Rifampin and rifapentine greatly reduce the concentrations of many antiretroviral agents; a less pronounced reduction is seen with rifabutin.[25] The rifamycins are metabolized by esterases to desacetylated derivatives. Although rifampin and rifapentine are not CYP substrates, the rifamycins are capable of autoinduction, showing a reduced AUC with repeated administration.[26]

Rifampin generally is well tolerated. Clinically relevant adverse effects include nausea, rash, and occasional hepatotoxicity. Rifampin-induced hepatitis occurs in up to 2.5% of patients treated with multidrug regimens, and it does not seem to be dose related.[27] The flulike syndrome is uncommon, and occurs most often with higher rifampin doses (1200 mg or more) given once or twice weekly.[28,29] Higher daily doses of rifampin seem to avoid the flulike syndrome. The rifamycins are potent inducers of CYP450 enzymes and several other enzymes and transporters, leading to numerous drug interactions. For example, clarithromycin concentrations are reduced by 50% with rifabutin and 90% by rifampin.[30]

Rifabutin is structurally similar to rifampin, but is more lipid soluble.[31] The increased lipid solubility results in a larger volume of distribution and slower clearance. Rifabutin's terminal half-life is approximately 37 hours. A 300-mg dose of rifabutin produces a C_{max} of 0.3 to 0.9 μg/mL (30-fold lower than rifampin) approximately 3 hours after the dose. Food does not affect rifabutin's C_{max} or AUC, but may cause a delay in absorption.[32]

In our experience, rifabutin is not well tolerated by many patients with NTM. Griffith and colleagues[33] noted similar results in patients with MAC treated with a thrice-weekly regimen of clarithromycin, ethambutol, and rifabutin. Twenty-four of 59 patients required a dose decrease or removal of the drug because of adverse effects.[33] In addition, rifabutin is a CYP3A4 substrate, resulting in bidirectional interactions. Important examples include clarithromycin and the azoles.[30,34]

Unlike rifampin, rifabutin is subject to concentration-related adverse effects. The risk of uveitis, leukopenia, and arthralgia increases with increasing concentrations. In general, high rifabutin concentrations are caused by the presence of a CYP inhibitor. For example, in a study of patients with HIV on a multidrug regimen of clarithromycin, rifabutin, and ethambutol, clarithromycin concentrations were decreased by rifabutin's enzyme induction, and rifabutin concentrations were increased because of clarithromycin inhibition.[35] Ritonavir and cobicistat can also increase rifabutin concentrations. Whenever a rifamycin is used, the clinician should examine the patient's maintenance medications, including antihypertensives, antiepileptics, and so forth, for additional drug-drug interactions.[36,37]

Rifapentine, a cyclopentyl derivative of rifampin, is approved for tuberculosis (TB) treatment. To date, it has not been studied for use in patients with NTM.

ETHAMBUTOL

Ethambutol's antimicrobial activity is limited to mycobacteria. It may be used for slow-growing NTM; rapidly growing NTM normally show high levels of resistance. Daily doses typically are 15 to 25 mg/kg, and produce a C_{max} of 2–6 μg/mL 2–3 hours after the dose.[38] For Mtb, intermittent doses (2 times weekly) as high as 50 mg/kg are used.

Optic neuritis is the most common adverse effect seen with ethambutol. Elderly patients and young patients with decreased renal function are at an increased risk because of reduced clearance. Snellen eye charts are used to test for visual acuity, whereas Ishihara color plates are used for red-green color discrimination. Patients should be tested at baseline and periodically during treatment. Increased serum uric acid values are occasionally seen with ethambutol. Drug interactions with ethambutol are uncommon.

FLUOROQUINOLONES

Ciprofloxacin, levofloxacin, and moxifloxacin are sometimes used for NTM infections. However, their role is not well established. For example, it is unclear whether the fluoroquinolones, when combined with macrolides, are able to prevent the selection of macrolide-resistant NTM. The fluoroquinolones show concentration-dependent killing of most bacteria and Mtb.

Ciprofloxacin doses of 500–750 mg (once or twice daily) produce a C_{max} of 4 to 6 μg/mL about 2 hours after the dose. Levofloxacin doses of 750–1000 mg once daily produce a C_{max} range of 8 to 12 μg/mL about 2 hours after the dose. Moxifloxacin doses of 400 mg daily produce a C_{max} of 3 to 5 μg/mL about 2 hours after the dose. Higher doses (600–800 mg daily) are being studied in patients with TB, but dose escalation must be done cautiously because of the risk of QT prolongation.[39] All 3 fluoroquinolones show extensive tissue penetration. Levofloxacin is renally cleared, whereas ciprofloxacin and moxifloxacin are cleared both renally and hepatically.

QT prolongation is the most serious class of adverse event requiring monitoring. Central nervous system adverse effects (headache, dizziness) and phototoxicity may occur. Tendinopathy also occurs with fluoroquinolone use.[40,41] Fluoroquinolones have a black-box warning regarding tendon rupture.[42] Risk factors for tendon rupture include advanced age (>60 years old), renal insufficiency, steroid use, type II diabetes, and a prior history of musculoskeletal disorders.[40,43] As with many antibiotics, patients should be warned of GI adverse effects such as nausea/vomiting and diarrhea.[44]

Drug interactions are not common with the fluoroquinolones. It is best not to administer fluoroquinolones within 2 hours of drugs, supplements, or foods containing divalent or trivalent cations because this may lead to the formation of insoluble chelating complexes and poor absorption of the fluoroquinolones.[45,46] Rifampin and rifapentine reduce moxifloxacin serum concentrations by 20% to 30%.[47–49] Increasing the moxifloxacin dose from 400 to 600 mg followed by TDM should be considered when moxifloxacin is coadministered with a rifamycin. Diabetic patients prescribed fluoroquinolones should monitor their glucose concentrations. In 2006, gatifloxacin was withdrawn from the market because of concerns over both hypoglycemic and hyperglycemic events.[50] Drug-induced dysglycemia has been associated with many of the remaining fluoroquinolones.[51]

AMINOGLYCOSIDES

Aminoglycosides show concentration-dependent killing of bacteria and mycobacteria. As a class, the aminoglycosides have similar pharmacokinetic profiles.[52] Amikacin and streptomycin are administered either intravenously or by intramuscular injection. Intravenous infusions can be given over 30 minutes.[53] Intramuscular injections typically are absorbed between 30 to 90 minutes. Typical aminoglycosides doses are 15 mg/kg daily, or 25 mg/kg when administered twice or thrice weekly. Smaller doses reduce the C_{max}, and may reduce efficacy. Linear regression is used to back-calculate to the end of the infusion and determine the C_{max}. As an alternative, Bayesian pharmacokinetic programs may be used. Daily doses produce a calculated C_{max} of 35 to 45 µg/mL (back-calculated to 1 hour

after intramuscular doses, or to the end of the intravenous infusion), whereas intermittent dosing produces a C_{max} of 65 to 80 µg/mL.[21] Elimination is by glomerular filtration, and doses need to be adjusted in patients with renal insufficiency. Elimination half-lives are 2 to 4 hours, depending on renal function. No metabolites have been identified thus far.

The primary clinical concerns with the aminoglycosides are auditory, vestibular, or nephrotoxicity. In a prospective study by Peloquin and colleagues,[54] toxicity was not related to either the size of the dose or the frequency of administration. An increased risk of ototoxicity was associated with older age and a larger cumulative dose.[54] It is common practice at some centers to reduce the dose to 10 mg/kg in older patients. However, this may be counterproductive. It may reduce efficacy without changing toxicity, which could prolong treatment, leading to a higher risk of toxicity in the longer term.

Drug interactions are minimal, because the aminoglycosides are not substrates or inducers/inhibitors of CYP enzymes. However, concurrent use with other potential nephrotoxins (eg, amphotericin B) may lead to additive nephrotoxicity.

CLOFAZIMINE

Clofazimine is best known for its role in the treatment of leprosy (caused by *Mycobacterium leprae* and possibly *Mycobacterium lepromatosis*). It has been used occasionally in the treatment of NTM infections. MICs range from 0.06 to 2 µg/mL, with many of the rapidly growing mycobacteria showing MICs of less than or equal to 1 µg/mL.[55,56] Its mechanism of action is not completely known. It may inhibit mycobacterial replication by binding to the guanine base of DNA.[57]

Clofazimine became less favored for NTM when a clinical study found that clofazimine plus clarithromycin and ethambutol was associated with increased mortality in disseminated MAC infections in patients with AIDS.[58] Clofazimine's use for other NTM infections remains poorly documented. In vitro studies show evidence that clofazimine may act synergistically with amikacin against rapidly growing NTM species.[56] However, this action remains to be demonstrated clinically. In addition, clofazimine can be difficult to obtain. In the United States, clinicians must submit an individual investigational new drug application to the FDA. In addition, cross-resistance between bedaquiline and clofazimine has been reported.[59] In vitro tests indicate that bedaquiline could be a potent NTM antibiotic, although that also remains to be demonstrated clinically.

Clofazimine is highly lipophilic, and it displays a long terminal half-life. Clofazimine is administered orally, most often at 100 mg daily. T_{max} normally is observed at 2 to 3 hours, but may be highly variable. Typical serum concentrations range from 0.5 to 2 μg/mL. Absorption is increased with food.

The most common adverse effect with clofazimine is a dose-related hyperpigmentation of body tissues.[60] This discoloration is visible within the first month of therapy, resulting in a tanning or bronzing effect seen in most individuals. Patients should be counseled that this bronze discoloration can last for a year following discontinuation of the drug. Drying of the skin may occur, but usually responds to the use of skin moisturizers. Photosensitivity may occur, so patients should use sunscreen and hats, and should avoid sun exposure when possible. Discoloration of the eye caused by crystalline deposits within the cornea and conjunctiva also can occur.[61] Crystal deposition may cause severe GI effects, necessitating discontinuation of the drug.[62] Drug interactions are uncommon.

LINEZOLID

An oxazolididione, linezolid, has activity against a large number of gram-positive bacteria, including many mycobacteria, such as Mtb and NTM.[63] Linezolid binds to the 23S subunit of a bacterium's ribosome to prevent protein synthesis.[64] MIC values range from 0.5 to 4 μg/mL for Mtb and most gram-positive cocci.[64,65] MICs are variable for NTM species.[64] In vitro testing of 53 clinical isolates showed that M abscessus and Mycobacterium intracellulare were the least susceptible to linezolid, whereas M avium and Mycobacterium gordonae were the most susceptible.[66] However, data are limited regarding linezolid's clinical efficacy.

Oral linezolid is completely absorbed, with bioavailability close to 100%. The dose for mycobacteria has not been established clearly. Empirical, once-daily dosing has been tried. The standard dose for gram-positive bacteria is 600 mg twice daily, and this produces C_{max} of 12 to 26 μg/mL 1 to 2 hours after the dose. C_{max} decreases approximately 17% when linezolid is taken with food, but AUC is unaffected.[67] Linezolid has good tissue penetration, producing concentrations higher than the MIC.[68] The drug has an elimination half-life of about 4 to 6 hours.

Linezolid may be considered for NTM infections, especially in cases in which organisms are resistant to primary choices.[69] Linezolid use is limited by its long-term adverse effects, including myelosuppression, ocular and peripheral neuropathy, and lactic acidosis. In a review by Narita and colleagues,[70] optic neuropathy resolved in those patients who stopped linezolid, but those experiencing peripheral neuropathy did not fully recover. The exact mechanisms through which these toxicities occur is not certain, but mitochondrial damage is strongly suspected.[71]

Linezolid is a weak monoamine oxidase inhibitor and increases the risk of serotonin toxicity (serotonin syndrome) when combined with additional serotonergic agents.[72] Although the incidence is small, clinicians should be aware of the potential interaction. Concurrent use of linezolid with rifampin may reduce linezolid serum concentrations. Two other oxazolidinones, AZD-5847 and PNU-100480 (sutezolid), are currently being investigated for use in TB treatment. Their roles for NTM infections currently are not known.

ISONIAZID

Aside from Mtb, isoniazid's (INH) coverage of mycobacteria is limited. Isoniazid's MIC range is 0.01 to 0.25 μg/mL for Mtb.[73,74] Among the NTM, Mycobacterium xenopi and M kansasii are susceptible, but M kansasii typically requires higher INH concentrations.

Isoniazid is a prodrug, converted by the enzyme katG within mycobacteria to its active form. The INH intermediates that are formed interfere with mycolic acid synthesis, disrupting the bacterial cell wall.[75] Organisms without katG display INH resistance. A C_{max} of 3 to 5 μg/mL is seen with 300 mg oral doses, whereas a C_{max} of 9 to 15 μg/mL is achieved with intermittent (2–3 times weekly) 900-mg doses. Isoniazid generally is well absorbed, although high-fat meals reduce isoniazid's C_{max} by 50%.[76] T_{max} typically is 1 to 2 hours after the dose, but may be delayed with a high-fat meal.[76] Isoniazid is widely distributed with a volume of distribution around 0.7 L/kg.[76] Isoniazid is metabolized by the liver to inactive metabolites, primarily by acetylation via N-acetyl transferase 2. Isoniazid's half-life in slow acetylators is between 3 and 4 hours, whereas for fast acetylators the half-life is less than 2 hours. Hepatotoxicity occurs in a small percentage of patients taking isoniazid. Chronic alcohol intake, age greater than 35 years, preexisting hepatic disease, and the concurrent use of other hepatotoxins are all considered risk factors. Isoniazid inhibits CYP450 enzymes, including CYP3A4 and CYP2C19, and may inhibit or induce CYP2E1.[77,78] In particular, the antiepileptics carbamazepine and phenytoin may have significant increases in plasma concentrations.[79,80] Clinicians should monitor patients for signs of toxicity (eg, ataxia, nystagmus) and routinely measure drug concentrations if concurrent use cannot be avoided.[80]

TIGECYCLINE

Tigecycline is a glycylcycline, specifically designed to avoid the resistance seen with the tetracyclines.[81] As with the tetracyclines, tigecycline binds to the bacterium's 30S ribosomal subunit and prevents protein synthesis.[82] Tigecycline is FDA approved for skin/soft tissue infections, as well as complicated intra-abdominal infections.[83] It has shown promise against the rapidly growing mycobacteria. Tigecycline has a reported MIC range between 0.06 and 0.25 µg/mL for M chelonae and M fortuitum, and 0.06 to 1 µg/mL for M abscessus.[84] Wallace and colleagues[85] reported favorable results when tigecycline was used as salvage treatment in patients with M abscessus and M chelonae. However, 90% of the patients experienced significant GI effects (nausea and vomiting), and less than half of the patients received the recommended dose of 100 mg daily. The average dose was not described. In this study, the use of antiemetic drugs became routine. Even though the manufacturer's recommended dose is 50 mg, in our experience some patients cannot tolerate even 25 mg of tigecycline daily without pretreatment with an antiemetic. The requirement for intravenous dosing also limits its appeal. Dosing for bacterial infections is every 12 hours. The frequency of dosing for NTM is less certain but, in the recent study described earlier, many patients improved on once-daily dosing.

Tigecycline is extensively distributed, with a volume of distribution between 7 and 10 L/kg.[86] The half-life has a wide range, caused by variability in the volume of distribution.[87] This variability may reflect nonlinear binding in the plasma or tissue.[87] C_{max} following a 1-hour infusion is about 1 µg/mL.

As noted, GI adverse effects are the primary complaint of most patients.[85] Tolerability may be improved by slowly increasing the dose and the use of antiemetics. Other adverse effects include photosensitivity, drug-induced hepatitis, risk of pancreatitis, and tooth discoloration in young children (as seen with other tetracyclines). In addition, the FDA reported an increased risk of death with tigecycline compared with other drugs used to treat serious skin and intra-abdominal infections. It carries a black-box warning for this reason.[16] However, there are conflicting studies regarding this warning statement.[88–90] Drug interactions with tigecycline are rare. Concurrent use of tigecycline with warfarin showed an increase in warfarin's AUC, but did not have a significant impact on International Normalized Ratio (INR).[83]

CEFOXITIN

Cefoxitin occasionally is used for treating NTM infections, particularly rapidly growing NTM.[91] Cefoxitin works by binding to penicillin-binding proteins (PBPs) that interfere with bacterial cell wall synthesis. Cefoxitin usually is administered intravenously to patients with NTM. Specific dosing for NTM species has not been established. Some clinicians recommend 1 to 2 g every 6 hours.[92] Cefoxitin has a half-life of about 45 minutes. Cefoxitin is renally eliminated, and dosage should be adjusted in patients with renal dysfunction.[91] Cefoxitin generally is well tolerated. GI adverse effects and local injection site reactions are the most common toxicities. High doses of β-lactams can, rarely, cause seizures.[91,93] Drug interactions with cefoxitin are rare. Probenecid increases cefoxitin serum concentrations through competitively inhibiting tubular secretion.[91] Patients taking warfarin may experience an increase in INR when used concurrently with cefoxitin.[91]

IMIPENEM

Like cefoxitin, imipenem occasionally is used to treat NTM infections. For M chelonae, imipenem is preferred because M chelonae is resistant to cefoxitin.[94,95] Imipenem binds to PBPs and interferes with bacterial cell wall synthesis. Imipenem is administered intravenously. Specific dosing for NTM species has not been established. Some clinicians recommend 500 mg 2 to 4 times daily.[96] Imipenem has a half-life of about 1 hour.[97] Adverse effects include GI and injection site reactions. In addition, imipenem has the potential for causing seizures that exceeds that of other β-lactams.[98] Drug interactions are rare. Similar to cefoxitin, imipenem may interact with probenecid and warfarin.[97] In addition, imipenem should be used cautiously with cyclosporine, ganciclovir, theophylline, and valproic acid.[97]

MONITORING DRUG TOXICITY DURING TREATMENT

As discussed by van Ingen and colleagues elsewhere in this issue, sputum microbiology remains the gold standard for monitoring the response to treatment of pulmonary NTM infections. However, many patients with NTM cannot produce an adequate sputum specimen for the initial diagnosis, and most stop producing sputum at some point during the course of effective treatment. TDM can help clinicians determine the best doses for drugs by revealing poor or delayed drug absorption or lack of adherence, and by untangling serious drug interactions. When tested (primarily with Mtb), antimycobacterial drug efficacy clearly is concentration dependent. Some adverse effects, such as ethambutol ocular toxicity, are also concentration dependent, so a clear rationale can be set forth for measuring and adjusting doses based on serum concentrations (**Table 1**). Otherwise, clinicians lack direct control over the drug therapy. In practice, obtaining TDM can be challenging, including issues related to preauthorization and medical insurance coverage, and related to logistical issues for patients who may need to travel considerable distances to have the samples collected.

Parameters for the clinical monitoring of adverse drug effects are shown in **Table 2**. The current ATS-IDSA guidelines on the management of NTM infections recommend monitoring for adverse drug reactions periodically, routinely, or at repeat intervals.[96] The exception is monitoring for ethambutol-induced optic neuritis, with monthly testing of visual acuity and color vision. This recommendation seems to be borrowed from guidelines for managing TB.[90] Some TB guidelines suggest monitoring for hepatotoxicity monthly; every 2 months; or at months 1, 3, and

6. However, those guidelines also review the lack of clinical trial evidence showing a benefit from such monitoring.[99] There is no definitive study regarding the optimal frequency of monitoring of patients with NTM for adverse drug reactions. Unlike patients with TB, patients with NTM do not receive directly observed therapy, and patients with NTM tend to be treated for much long periods of time. Our compromise in the University of Florida NTM Clinic has been to monitor blood tests (eg, cell blood count, liver function tests) every 3 months in patients without symptoms of adverse reactions. We also suggest this period for monitoring of visual acuity and color vision, or a professional eye examination if patients have no visual symptoms. This approach seems to be logistically feasible and tolerable for most patients. However, we also educate patients at each visit to report any new symptoms that may be adverse events; adverse events can occur during the intervals of monitoring tests.

Common serious adverse drug reactions include ototoxicity from the aminoglycosides. Amikacin often is added for cavitary MAC infections, or for *M abscessus* group infections. Unlike streptomycin, amikacin serum concentrations are easy to obtain. Peripherally inserted central catheters are well used in patients with NTM, given the long durations of treatment. Baseline serum blood urea nitrogen (BUN) and serum creatinine levels can be checked as often as weekly to observe for nephrotoxicity. Serum amikacin concentrations are described earlier. Baseline and periodic audiology evaluations are advisable on all patients who receive either systemic or inhaled amikacin. Many patients with NTM are elderly, and they frequently have mild baseline hearing loss or tinnitus. Such patients may require more frequent audiometry. Patients should be instructed to call their clinicians immediately with any symptoms of increasing tinnitus, decreased hearing, unsteadiness of gait, vertigo, or lightheadedness. We aim to obtain audiometry at baseline and after 2 weeks of intravenous amikacin. If it is stable and there are no other symptoms, monthly audiometry is reasonable. Testing for vestibular toxicity can be performed with a Romberg test, ideally while the patient is standing on compliant foam. Additional tests are available.[100,101]

Optic neuritis caused by ethambutol is a toxicity that many clinicians and patients seem to fear out of proportion to its true incidence. Current NTM guidelines suggest monitoring for toxicity at monthly visits. Although it may seem intuitive that monitoring monthly would be more sensitive in detecting toxicity, we are not aware of data to support that practice. We ask our patients to have their

Table 1
Targeted maximum drug concentrations for TDM

Drug	Dose	Concentration Target Range (µg/mL)
Clarithromycin	500 mg	2–7
Azithromycin	500 mg	0.2–0.7
Amikacin (daily)	15 mg/kg	35–45[a]
Streptomycin (daily)	15 mg/kg	34–45[a]
Rifampin	600 mg	8–24
Rifabutin	300 mg	0.3–0.9
Ciprofloxacin	750 mg	4–6
Levofloxacin	750–1000 mg	8–12
Moxifloxacin	400 mg	3–5
Ethambutol	20 mg/kg	2–6
Linezolid	600 mg	12–26
Isoniazid (daily)	300 mg	3–5
Tigecycline	25–50 mg	1

[a] Back-calculated to end of infusion or 1 hour after intramuscular dose.

Table 2
Monitoring parameters

Drug	Adverse Events	Monitoring Parameters	Comment
Clarithromycin	GI, QT prolongation	EKG, LFTs Baseline audiogram	CYP3A4 inhibitor
Azithromycin	GI, QT prolongation	EKG, LFTs Baseline audiogram	—
Aminoglycosides	Vestibular/auditory, renal	BUN, SCr Audiometry Romberg test	Caution when using with other potential nephrotoxins. Monitor renal function. Monitor for auditory and vestibular toxicity
Rifampin	Hepatotoxicity, flulike syndrome	CBC, LFTs	Potent enzyme inducer May monitor renal function
Rifabutin	Uveitis	CBC, LFTs	—
Ciprofloxacin	GI, tendonitis, QT prolongation	EKG	—
Levofloxacin	GI, tendonitis, QT prolongation	EKG	—
Moxifloxacin	GI, tendonitis, QT prolongation	EKG	—
Ethambutol	Optic neuritis	Baseline eye examination Snellen eye chart Ishihara color plates	Baseline color vision and visual acuity should be conducted at initial visit and each month thereafter
Linezolid	Neuropathy Thrombocytopenia, myelosuppression Optic neuritis	Symptoms CBC Eye examinations Snellen eye chart, Ishihara color plates	—
Isoniazid	Liver, peripheral neuropathy	LFTs	Administer with pyridoxine
Tigecycline	GI	LFTs Amylase, lipase	—
Cefoxitin	GI, seizures	CBC, LFTs, renal function	Cannot replace with other cephalosporins
Imipenem	GI, seizures	CBC, LFTs, renal function	—

Abbreviations: BUN, blood urea nitrogen; CBC, complete blood count; EKG, electrocardiogram; LFTs, liver function tests; SCr, serum creatinine.

vision checked with at least a Snellen vision chart and Ishihara color plates at least every 3 months. This testing can be done with their primary care physicians or with their eye care specialists, as they choose, and usually results in patients being seen about every 6 to 8 weeks. We educate patients about optic neuritis and ask that they stop the ethambutol and call us, or their eye clinician, if there is any question of a change in vision, and we review this at every visit. This practice has usually resulted in the detection of eye diseases other than optic neuritis. The 3-month interval also seems to be an appropriate frequency to monitor the complete blood count for rifampin, imipenem or tigecycline toxicity, and liver function tests to detect drug-induced hepatitis from rifampin, the macrolides, imipenem, or tigecycline. Serum BUN and creatinine levels can be used to assess renal function, as needed. Although uncommon, renal function changes induced by rifampin or β-lactam can occur. We also test amylase and lipase levels for patients on tigecycline and renal function for patients on imipenem. This interval is also the frequency at which we prefer to follow our patients in the clinic, so logistically they are reminded to have their monitoring done before the clinic visit.

Although we are not aware of clinically significant QT prolongation causing life-threatening arrhythmias in a patient with NTM, there has been increasing concern about QT prolongation with macrolides and we are now being more attentive to this risk.[15,102] We generally ask patients to provide us with a recent electrocardiogram (EKG); if not available then we obtain a baseline EKG. We then repeat the EKG 1 to 2 weeks after initiation of macrolide therapy to rule out significant QT prolongation.

We have found that the best way to avoid drug-drug interactions with both rifabutin and clarithromycin is simply to avoid using those drugs. We concur with the NTM guidelines that most patients with NTM, especially elderly women, do not tolerate rifabutin. Azithromycin generally is well tolerated, and its serum concentrations are less affected by rifampin than are those of clarithromycin. Some patients who tolerate clarithromycin better than azithromycin do so because they have very low drug concentrations, because of the interaction with rifampin. The macrolides also have been associated rarely with hearing loss, so we prefer to obtain a baseline audiology consultation given the anticipated long duration of treatment. We only repeat the audiometry if there are new symptoms suggesting ototoxicity.

There is a need for evidence to support specific monitoring of drug toxicities, and we suggest that this be studied in future clinical trials. Operational research also could evaluate the use of self-monitoring. In the modern age of smart phones, there are new applications for testing of both vision and hearing that could be used as screening tools by patients.

SUMMARY/DISCUSSION

The treatment of NTM infections is long, challenging, and sometimes ineffective. Data specific to the treatment of NTM infections, including detailed pharmacokinetic/pharmacodynamic data, are lacking. The drugs used are borrowed from the treatments of other types of infections, and data from large, prospective randomized trials to guide treatments are lacking. Thus, the data presented here can only be seen as suggestions based on current empirical evidence and clinical experience. It is hoped that in the future NTM-specific drugs will be dosed based on clinical trial data.

REFERENCES

1. Runyon EH. Identification of mycobacterial pathogens utilizing colony characteristics. Am J Clin Pathol 1970;54:578–86.
2. Nie W, Duan H, Huang H, et al. Species identification of *Mycobacterium abscessus* subsp. *abscessus* and *Mycobacterium abscessus* subsp. *bolletii* using rpoB and hsp65, and susceptibility testing to eight antibiotics. Int J Infect Dis 2014;25:170–4.
3. Chaisson RE, Benson CA, Dube MP, et al. Clarithromycin therapy for bacteremic *Mycobacterium avium* complex disease. A randomized, double-blind, dose-ranging study in patients with AIDS. AIDS Clinical Trials Group Protocol 157 Study Team. Ann Intern Med 1994;121:905–11.
4. Mangoni AA, Jackson SH. Age-related changes in pharmacokinetics and pharmacodynamics: basic principles and practical applications. Br J Clin Pharmacol 2004;57:6–14.
5. Nash KA, Zhang Y, Brown-Elliott BA, et al. Molecular basis of intrinsic macrolide resistance in clinical isolates of *Mycobacterium fortuitum*. J Antimicrob Chemother 2005;55:170–7.
6. Meier A, Heifets L, Wallace RJ Jr, et al. Molecular mechanisms of clarithromycin resistance in *Mycobacterium avium*: observation of multiple 23S rDNA mutations in a clonal population. J Infect Dis 1996;174:354–60.
7. Meier A, Kirschner P, Springer B, et al. Identification of mutations in 23S rRNA gene of clarithromycin-resistant *Mycobacterium intracellulare*. Antimicrob Agents Chemother 1994;38:381–4.
8. Zuckerman JM. Macrolides and ketolides: azithromycin, clarithromycin, telithromycin. Infect Dis Clin North Am 2004;18:621–49, xi.
9. Biaxin [Package Insert]. North Chicago, IL: Inc A; 2013.
10. Zithromax [package insert]. New York, NY: Inc P; 2014.
11. Whitman MS, Tunkel AR. Azithromycin and clarithromycin: overview and comparison with erythromycin. Infect Control Hosp Epidemiol 1992;13:357–68.
12. Maisch NM, Kochupurackal JG, Sin J. Azithromycin and the risk of cardiovascular complications. J Pharm Pract 2014;27:496–500.
13. Milberg P, Eckardt L, Bruns HJ, et al. Divergent proarrhythmic potential of macrolide antibiotics despite similar QT prolongation: fast phase 3 repolarization prevents early afterdepolarizations and torsade de pointes. J Pharmacol Exp Ther 2002;303:218–25.
14. Volberg WA, Koci BJ, Su W, et al. Blockade of human cardiac potassium channel human ether-a-go-go-related gene (HERG) by macrolide antibiotics. J Pharmacol Exp Ther 2002;302:320–7.
15. Ray WA, Murray KT, Hall K, et al. Azithromycin and the risk of cardiovascular death. N Engl J Med 2012;366:1881–90.
16. FDA Drug Safety Communication. Azithromycin (Zithromax or Zmax) and the risk of potentially fatal heart rhythms. 2013. Available at: http://www.fda.gov/drugs/drugsafety/ucm341822.htm. Accessed August 27, 2014.

17. Svanstrom H, Pasternak B, Hviid A. Use of clarithromycin and roxithromycin and risk of cardiac death: cohort study. BMJ 2014;349:g4930.

18. Wong E, Nguyen TV. A case-based approach to evaluating azithromycin use and cardiovascular risks. Consult Pharm 2014;29:47–52.

19. Wehrli W. Rifampin: mechanisms of action and resistance. Rev Infect Dis 1983;5(Suppl 3): S407–11.

20. Gumbo T, Louie A, Deziel MR, et al. Concentration-dependent *Mycobacterium tuberculosis* killing and prevention of resistance by rifampin. Antimicrob Agents Chemother 2007;51:3781–8.

21. Peloquin CA. Therapeutic drug monitoring of the antimycobacterial drugs. Clin Lab Med 1996;16: 717–29.

22. Peloquin CA, Namdar R, Singleton MD, et al. Pharmacokinetics of rifampin under fasting conditions, with food, and with antacids. Chest 1999;115:12–8.

23. Peloquin CA, Nitta AT, Burman WJ, et al. Low antituberculosis drug concentrations in patients with AIDS. Ann Pharmacother 1996;30:919–25.

24. Gilljam M, Berning SE, Peloquin CA, et al. Therapeutic drug monitoring in patients with cystic fibrosis and mycobacterial disease. Eur Respir J 1999;14:347–51.

25. Regazzi M, Carvalho AC, Villani P, et al. Treatment optimization in patients co-infected with HIV and mycobacterium tuberculosis infections: focus on drug-drug interactions with rifamycins. Clin Pharmacokinet 2014;53:489–507.

26. Strolin Benedetti M, Dostert P. Induction and auto-induction properties of rifamycin derivatives: a review of animal and human studies. Environ Health Perspect 1994;102(Suppl 9):101–5.

27. Long MW, Snider DE Jr, Farer LS. U.S. Public Health Service Cooperative trial of three rifampin-isoniazid regimens in treatment of pulmonary tuberculosis. Am Rev Respir Dis 1979;119:879–94.

28. A comparative study of daily followed by twice or once weekly regimens of ethambutol and rifampicin in retreatment of patients with pulmonary tuberculosis. The results at 1 year. A cooperative tuberculosis chemotherapy study in Poland. Tubercle 1975;56:1–26.

29. Burman WJ, Gallicano K, Peloquin C. Comparative pharmacokinetics and pharmacodynamics of the rifamycin antibacterials. Clin Pharmacokinet 2001; 40:327–41.

30. Wallace RJ Jr, Brown BA, Griffith DE, et al. Reduced serum levels of clarithromycin in patients treated with multidrug regimens including rifampin or rifabutin for *Mycobacterium avium-M. intracellulare* infection. J Infect Dis 1995;171:747–50.

31. Blaschke TF, Skinner MH. The clinical pharmacokinetics of rifabutin. Clin Infect Dis 1996;22(Suppl 1): S15–21 [discussion: S21–2].

32. Narang PK, Lewis RC, Bianchine JR. Rifabutin absorption in humans: relative bioavailability and food effect. Clin Pharmacol Ther 1992;52:335–41.

33. Griffith DE, Brown BA, Cegielski P, et al. Early results (at 6 months) with intermittent clarithromycin-including regimens for lung disease due to *Mycobacterium avium* complex. Clin Infect Dis 2000;30: 288–92.

34. Schwiesow JN, Iseman MD, Peloquin CA. Concomitant use of voriconazole and rifabutin in a patient with multiple infections. Pharmacotherapy 2008; 28:1076–80.

35. Hafner R, Bethel J, Power M, et al. Tolerance and pharmacokinetic interactions of rifabutin and clarithromycin in human immunodeficiency virus-infected volunteers. Antimicrob Agents Chemother 1998;42:631–9.

36. Egelund EF, Fennelly KP, Peloquin CP. Concomitant use of carbamazepine and rifampin in a patient with *Mycobacterium avium* complex and seizure disorder. J Pharm Technol 2014;30:93–6.

37. Yoshimoto H, Takahashi M, Saima S. Influence of rifampicin on antihypertensive effects of dihydropiridine calcium-channel blockers in four elderly patients. Nihon Ronen Igakkai Zasshi 1996;33:692–6 [in Japanese].

38. Griffith DE, Brown-Elliott BA, Shepherd S, et al. Ethambutol ocular toxicity in treatment regimens for *Mycobacterium avium* complex lung disease. Am J Respir Crit Care Med 2005;172:250–3.

39. Demolis JL, Kubitza D, Tenneze L, et al. Effect of a single oral dose of moxifloxacin (400 mg and 800 mg) on ventricular repolarization in healthy subjects. Clin Pharmacol Ther 2000;68:658–66.

40. Kim GK. The risk of fluoroquinolone-induced tendinopathy and tendon rupture: what does the clinician need to know? J Clin Aesthet Dermatol 2010; 3:49–54.

41. Corrao G, Zambon A, Bertu L, et al. Evidence of tendinitis provoked by fluoroquinolone treatment: a case-control study. Drug Saf 2006;29: 889–96.

42. Tanne JH. FDA adds "black box" warning label to fluoroquinolone antibiotics. BMJ 2008;337:a816.

43. Yu C, Giuffre B. Achilles tendinopathy after treatment with fluoroquinolone. Australas Radiol 2005; 49:407–10.

44. Fitton A. The quinolones. An overview of their pharmacology. Clin Pharmacokinet 1992;22(Suppl 1): 1–11.

45. King DE, Malone R, Lilley SH. New classification and update on the quinolone antibiotics. Am Fam Physician 2000;61:2741–8.

46. Rodvold KA, Piscitelli SC. New oral macrolide and fluoroquinolone antibiotics: an overview of pharmacokinetics, interactions, and safety. Clin Infect Dis 1993;17(Suppl 1):S192–9.

47. Nijland HM, Ruslami R, Suroto AJ, et al. Rifampicin reduces plasma concentrations of moxifloxacin in patients with tuberculosis. Clin Infect Dis 2007;45: 1001–7.

48. Weiner M, Burman W, Luo CC, et al. Effects of rifampin and multidrug resistance gene polymorphism on concentrations of moxifloxacin. Antimicrob Agents Chemother 2007;51:2861–6.

49. Dooley K, Flexner C, Hackman J, et al. Repeated administration of high-dose intermittent rifapentine reduces rifapentine and moxifloxacin plasma concentrations. Antimicrob Agents Chemother 2008; 52:4037–42.

50. Aspinall SL, Good CB, Jiang R, et al. Severe dysglycemia with the fluoroquinolones: a class effect? Clin Infect Dis 2009;49:402–8.

51. Park-Wyllie LY, Juurlink DN, Kopp A, et al. Outpatient gatifloxacin therapy and dysglycemia in older adults. N Engl J Med 2006;354:1352–61.

52. Peloquin CA, editor. Antituberculosis drugs: pharmacokinetics. Boca Raton (FL): CRC Press; 1991.

53. Zhu M, Burman WJ, Jaresko GS, et al. Population pharmacokinetics of intravenous and intramuscular streptomycin in patients with tuberculosis. Pharmacotherapy 2001;21:1037–45.

54. Peloquin CA, Berning SE, Nitta AT, et al. Aminoglycoside toxicity: daily versus thrice-weekly dosing for treatment of mycobacterial diseases. Clin Infect Dis 2004;38:1538–44.

55. Reddy VM, Nadadhur G, Daneluzzi D, et al. Antituberculosis activities of clofazimine and its new analogs B4154 and B4157. Antimicrob Agents Chemother 1996;40:633–6.

56. van Ingen J, Totten SE, Helstrom NK, et al. In vitro synergy between clofazimine and amikacin in treatment of nontuberculous mycobacterial disease. Antimicrob Agents Chemother 2012;56:6324–7.

57. Arbiser JL, Moschella SL. Clofazimine: a review of its medical uses and mechanisms of action. J Am Acad Dermatol 1995;32:241–7.

58. Chaisson RE, Keiser P, Pierce M, et al. Clarithromycin and ethambutol with or without clofazimine for the treatment of bacteremic Mycobacterium avium complex disease in patients with HIV infection. AIDS 1997;11:311–7.

59. Hartkoorn RC, Uplekar S, Cole ST. Cross-resistance between clofazimine and bedaquiline through upregulation of MmpL5 in Mycobacterium tuberculosis. Antimicrob Agents Chemother 2014; 58:2979–81.

60. Alsultan A, Peloquin CA. Therapeutic drug monitoring in the treatment of tuberculosis: an update. Drugs 2014;74:839–54.

61. Kaur I, Ram J, Kumar B, et al. Effect of clofazimine on eye in multibacillary leprosy. Indian J Lepr 1990;62: 87–90.

62. Garrelts JC. Clofazimine: a review of its use in leprosy and Mycobacterium avium complex infection. DICP 1991;25:525–31.

63. Wallace RJ Jr, Brown-Elliott BA, Ward SC, et al. Activities of linezolid against rapidly growing mycobacteria. Antimicrob Agents Chemother 2001;45: 764–7.

64. Livermore DM. Linezolid in vitro: mechanism and antibacterial spectrum. J Antimicrob Chemother 2003;51(Suppl 2):ii9–16.

65. Rodriguez JC, Ruiz M, Lopez M, et al. In vitro activity of moxifloxacin, levofloxacin, gatifloxacin and linezolid against Mycobacterium tuberculosis. Int J Antimicrob Agents 2002;20:464–7.

66. Cavusoglu C, Soyler I, Akinci P. Activities of linezolid against nontuberculous mycobacteria. New Microbiol 2007;30:411–4.

67. Zyvox [Package Insert]. New York: Pfizer; 2011.

68. Gee T, Ellis R, Marshall G, et al. Pharmacokinetics and tissue penetration of linezolid following multiple oral doses. Antimicrob Agents Chemother 2001;45:1843–6.

69. Brown-Elliott BA, Wallace RJ Jr, Blinkhorn R, et al. Successful treatment of disseminated Mycobacterium chelonae infection with linezolid. Clin Infect Dis 2001;33:1433–4.

70. Narita M, Tsuji BT, Yu VL. Linezolid-associated peripheral and optic neuropathy, lactic acidosis, and serotonin syndrome. Pharmacotherapy 2007;27: 1189–97.

71. Kopterides P, Papadomichelakis E, Armaganidis A. Linezolid use associated with lactic acidosis. Scand J Infect Dis 2005;37:153–4.

72. Quinn DK, Stern TA. Linezolid and serotonin syndrome. Prim Care Companion J Clin Psychiatry 2009;11:353–6.

73. Verbist L. Mode of action of antituberculous drugs (part I). Medicon Intl 1974;3:11–23.

74. Verbist L. Mode of action of antituberculous drugs (parts II). Medicon Intl 1974;3:3–17.

75. Timmins GS, Deretic V. Mechanisms of action of isoniazid. Mol Microbiol 2006;62:1220–7.

76. Peloquin CA, Namdar R, Dodge AA, et al. Pharmacokinetics of isoniazid under fasting conditions, with food, and with antacids. Int J Tuberc Lung Dis 1999;3:703–10.

77. Zand R, Nelson SD, Slattery JT, et al. Inhibition and induction of cytochrome P4502E1-catalyzed oxidation by isoniazid in humans. Clin Pharmacol Ther 1993;54:142–9.

78. Desta Z, Soukhova NV, Flockhart DA. Inhibition of cytochrome P450 (CYP450) isoforms by isoniazid: potent inhibition of CYP2C19 and CYP3A. Antimicrob Agents Chemother 2001;45:382–92.

79. Brennan RW, Dehejia H, Kutt H, et al. Diphenylhydantoin intoxication attendant to slow inactivation of isoniazid. Neurology 1970;20:687–93.

80. Wright JM, Stokes EF, Sweeney VP. Isoniazid-induced carbamazepine toxicity and vice versa: a double drug interaction. N Engl J Med 1982;307: 1325–7.

81. Rose WE, Rybak MJ. Tigecycline: first of a new class of antimicrobial agents. Pharmacotherapy 2006;26:1099–110.

82. da Silva LM, Nunes Salgado HR. Tigecycline: a review of properties, applications, and analytical methods. Ther Drug Monit 2010;32:282–8.

83. Tygacil [package insert]. New York: Inc. P; 2014.

84. Stein GE, Craig WA. Tigecycline: a critical analysis. Clin Infect Dis 2006;43:518–24.

85. Wallace RJ Jr, Dukart G, Brown-Elliott BA, et al. Clinical experience in 52 patients with tigecycline-containing regimens for salvage treatment of Mycobacterium abscessus and Mycobacterium chelonae infections. J Antimicrob Chemother 2014;69:1945–53.

86. Muralidharan G, Micalizzi M, Speth J, et al. Pharmacokinetics of tigecycline after single and multiple doses in healthy subjects. Antimicrob Agents Chemother 2005;49:220–9.

87. Barbour A, Schmidt S, Ma B, et al. Clinical pharmacokinetics and pharmacodynamics of tigecycline. Clin Pharmacokinet 2009;48:575–84.

88. Yahav D, Lador A, Paul M, et al. Efficacy and safety of tigecycline: a systematic review and meta-analysis. J Antimicrob Chemother 2011;66: 1963–71.

89. Tasina E, Haidich AB, Kokkali S, et al. Efficacy and safety of tigecycline for the treatment of infectious diseases: a meta-analysis. Lancet Infect Dis 2011;11:834–44.

90. Cai Y, Wang R, Liang B, et al. Systematic review and meta-analysis of the effectiveness and safety of tigecycline for treatment of infectious disease. Antimicrob Agents Chemother 2011;55:1162–72.

91. Mefoxin [package insert]. Rockford, IL: Mylan Institutional L; 2013.

92. De Groote MA, Huitt G. Infections due to rapidly growing mycobacteria. Clin Infect Dis 2006;42: 1756–63.

93. Chow KM, Hui AC, Szeto CC. Neurotoxicity induced by beta-lactam antibiotics: from bench to bedside. Eur J Clin Microbiol Infect Dis 2005;24:649–53.

94. Swenson JM, Wallace RJ Jr, Silcox VA, et al. Antimicrobial susceptibility of five subgroups of Mycobacterium fortuitum and Mycobacterium chelonae. Antimicrob Agents Chemother 1985;28:807–11.

95. Wallace RJ Jr, Brown BA, Onyi GO. Skin, soft tissue, and bone infections due to Mycobacterium chelonae chelonae: importance of prior corticosteroid therapy, frequency of disseminated infections, and resistance to oral antimicrobials other than clarithromycin. J Infect Dis 1992;166:405–12.

96. Griffith DE, Aksamit T, Brown-Elliott BA, et al. An official ATS/IDSA statement: diagnosis, treatment, and prevention of nontuberculous mycobacterial diseases. Am J Respir Crit Care Med 2007;175: 367–416.

97. Primaxin [Package Insert]. Whitehouse Station, NJ: Merck & Co; 2012.

98. Eng RH, Munsif AN, Yangco BG, et al. Seizure propensity with imipenem. Arch Intern Med 1989;149: 1881–3.

99. American Thoracic Society, CDC, Infectious Diseases Society of America. Treatment of tuberculosis. MMWR Recomm Rep 2003;52:1–80.

100. Longridge NS, Mallinson AI. The dynamic illegible E-test: a technique for assessing the vestibulo-ocular reflex. Acta Otolaryngol 1987;103:273–9.

101. Schubert MC, Tusa RJ, Grine LE, et al. Optimizing the sensitivity of the head thrust test for identifying vestibular hypofunction. Phys Ther 2004;84:151–8.

102. Mosholder AD, Mathew J, Alexander JJ, et al. Cardiovascular risks with azithromycin and other antibacterial drugs. N Engl J Med 2013;368:1665–8.

The Treatment of Rapidly Growing Mycobacterial Infections

Shannon H. Kasperbauer, MD[a,b,*],
Mary Ann De Groote, MD[c]

KEYWORDS

- *Mycobacterium abscessus* • *Mycobacterium massiliense* • Antimicrobial therapy
- NTM lung diseases • Antimicrobial resistance • Drug susceptibility testing • Surgical therapy

KEY POINTS

- The *Mycobacterium abscessus* complex represent the most drug-resistant nontuberculous mycobacteria (NTM) and are the most difficult to treat.
- Treatment of rapidly growing mycobacterial infections is lengthy and expensive.
- Species-specific response to macrolides might explain improved outcomes in *M massiliense* lung disease.
- New drugs with bactericidal activity against NTM are needed.
- Preclinical in vivo testing models should mimic human disease presentation.

RAPIDLY GROWING MYCOBACTERIA AND NEW SEQUENCING TOOLS

Important pathogenic members of the rapidly growing mycobacteria (RGM) have undergone a series of taxonomic descriptions.[1–3] In the 1990s, many laboratories referred to the major RGM as *Mycobacterium chelonae* complex or *M fortuitum* complex until the appreciation that 2 major pathogens: *M abscessus* and *M chelonae* were unique. Although most clinicians have access to laboratories capable of identifying clinical isolates using the 16s rDNA sequencing, this methodology cannot reliably distinguish between these 2 closely related species. Later, we realized that *M abscessus* complex consisted of 3 subspecies: *M abscessus*, *M bolletii*, or *M massiliense*. However, currently a single official taxon unites *M massiliense* and *M bolletii* as *M abscessus* subsp. *bolletii*

and *M abscessus subsp. abscessus*. Fortunately, these species are undergoing taxonomic reevaluation. Modern genomic tools are revolutionizing microbiology and the use of whole-genome sequencing is becoming less expensive and more readily accessible. Using these highly discriminatory new genomic techniques, it has become clear that 3 subspecies of the *M abscessus* group should be considered a separate species.[4,5] In addition to specific identification, these high-throughput genome sequencing datasets have been extremely useful in understanding the epidemiology of RGM infections in outbreak settings[6] and in understanding strain-specific disease pathogenesis.[7] Whole-genome sequencing and molecular epidemiology have recently shed light on a large global "outbreak" of a highly related strain of *M massiliense* occurring in the UK, the

Disclosures: None.
[a] Division of Mycobacterial and Respiratory Infections, National Jewish Health, 1400 Jackson Street, Denver, CO 80206, USA; [b] Division of Infectious Diseases, University of Colorado Health Sciences Center, 12700 East 19th Avenue, Research Complex 2, Campus Box B168, Aurora, CO 80045, USA; [c] Department of Microbiology, Immunology and Pathology, Colorado State University, Campus Box 1682, Fort Collins, CO 80523, USA
* Corresponding author. National Jewish Health, 1400 Jackson Street, Denver, CO 80206.
E-mail address: Kasperbauers@njhealth.org

Clin Chest Med 36 (2015) 67–78
http://dx.doi.org/10.1016/j.ccm.2014.10.004
0272-5231/15/$ – see front matter © 2015 Elsevier Inc. All rights reserved.

United State, and Brazil.[8] Strains from 2 cystic fibrosis clinics showed high-level relatedness with each other and major-level relatedness with strains that caused soft tissue infections during an epidemic in Brazil. Many of the isolates were highly drug resistant.[9,10] More work is necessary to identify the mechanisms of spread of this conserved strain. We will see the use of whole-genome sequencing for some time to come.

DOES THE SPECIES MATTER FOR OUTCOMES OF DISEASE AND TREATMENT?

Genetic tools can also play a role in differentiating patients with heterogeneous clinical presentation and prognoses. For instance, utilizing a development cohort (48 isolates) and validation cohort (63 isolates), Shin and colleagues[11] looked at predicting disease phenotype (stable nodular bronchiectatic disease vs those who had progressive forms and fibrocavitary disease) based on a bacterial typing scheme called variable number of tandem repeat loci (**Figs. 1** and **2**). Others have also shown drug susceptibility differences and clinical outcome measures between M abscessus and M massiliense,[12] supporting the need to identify to the species level.

DRUG SUSCEPTIBILITY IN RAPIDLY GROWING MYCOBACTERIA

It is recommended that drug susceptibility testing for the RGM be performed by broth microdilution. The species of the M abscessus complex are typically more drug resistant compared with M chelonae and M fortuitum. M abscessus is resistant to

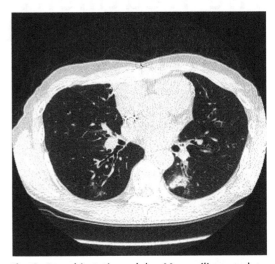

Fig. 2. Bronchiectatic nodular M massiliense pulmonary disease.

the first-line antituberculous mycobacterial agents, including rifampin, isoniazid, ethambutol, and pyrazinamide. In general, M abscessus is considered to be susceptible to amikacin, cefoxitin, and clarithromycin, and moderately susceptible to imipenem.[1] With the exception of the macrolide class, the correlation between in vitro susceptibility and clinical response for specific antimycobacterial drugs has not been established.[1,13] Therefore, the clinician should use the drug susceptibility report with an appreciation for its limitations.

A study from Korea reported drug susceptibility testing for 74 isolates of M abscessus.[14] Identification of the species was performed using the polymerase chain reaction-restriction fragment length polymorphism method based on the rpoB gene. Most of the isolates were found to be susceptible to amikacin (99%) and cefoxitin (99%). Amikacin had much better activity compared with tobramycin (36%). Imipenem was found to have activity against 55% of isolates. Clarithromycin showed activity in most isolates (91%) and the fluoroquinolones showed moderate activity with moxifloxacin (73%), seeming to be more active in vitro than ciprofloxacin (57%). Doxycycline was only susceptible in 7% of isolates. This was one of the few studies that noted such high rates of susceptibility for the quinolones.

A study of 102 isolates from Japan noted M abscessus and M massiliense showed an high level of resistance to all antimicrobials, except for clarithromycin, kanamycin, and amikacin.[12] Resistance to clarithromycin was more frequent in M abscessus than M massiliense (16% vs 4%, respectively).

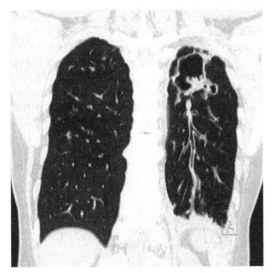

Fig. 1. Cavitary M abscessus pulmonary disease.

A report from China noted drug susceptibility in 210 isolates of M abscessus.[15] Amikacin was the most active drug among the agents tested (90%). Most isolates noted intermediate susceptibility to cefoxitin (87%) with only 9% susceptible. Of the isolates, 43% were susceptible to imipenem, 36% with intermediate susceptibility. Only 60% of the isolates were susceptible to clarithromycin, 26% with intermediate susceptibility. Susceptibility to ciprofloxacin and ofloxacin were low (3% and 4%, respectively). Moxifloxacin was not tested in this study.

An investigation from Taiwan of 40 clinical isolates of M abscessus noted susceptibility to amikacin (95%), cefoxitin (32%), ciprofloxacin (10%), clarithromycin (92.5%), doxycycline (7.5%), imipenem (12.5%), moxifloxacin (22.5%), sulfamethoxazole (7.5%), and tigecylcine (100%).[16]

Clofazimine (a riminophenazine) is a standard antimycobacterial agent used in leprosy which has excellent activity in vitro against the RGM. This agent is attractive because it has long half-life (65–70 days), slow metabolic elimination, and high concentration in macrophages and phagocytes.[17] A study from Taiwan noted susceptibility rates of 99.1%, 91.7%, and 100% in M abscessus, M fortuitum, and M chelonae isolates, respectively.[18] The authors also report synergism between clofazimine and amikacin in all of the M abscessus and M chelonae isolates tested. Synergy was also noted in an article by Van Ingen and colleagues.[19] In this study, 97% of the RGM had a minimum inhibitory concentration (MIC) of 1 μg/mL or less to clofazimine and 93% were susceptible to amikacin. The combination of clofazimine and amikacin proved to be synergistic in 82% of the M abscessus isolates with a 4- to 8-fold decrease in the MICs of both drugs.

Tigecycline is a glycylcycline with activity against the RGM.[20] The disadvantages are that tigecylcine is only available in an intravenous (IV) form and has high rates of associated nausea and vomiting. There are reports of clinical improvement with this agent, including cases of infection in immunocompromised individuals or as salvage therapy in cystic fibrosis.[21–23]

One reason for this lack of correlation between in vitro studies and clinical outcomes could be related to the differential antibiotic susceptibility of mycobacteria variants in biofilms and macrophages. M abscessus is in a stationary phase in the mature biofilm and 1 study showed that clarithromycin was relatively inactive against M abscessus in the biofilm.[24] These investigators also discovered that amikacin, cefoxitin, and clarithromycin were only bacteriostatic for M abscessus

variants at 10 times their MIC in a human macrophage model. These results suggest why it is so difficult to cure patients with M abscessus pulmonary disease.

MACROLIDE RESISTANCE

Macrolides function as antibiotics by binding to the 23S ribosomal RNA and blocking bacterial protein synthesis. Resistance to the macrolides has been described as arising from a point mutation in a region of the rrl gene encoding the peptidyltransferase domain of the 23S rRNA.[25] RGM have only a single chromosomal copy of the rRNA operon, thus making them susceptible to single-step mutations. Another method of resistance occurs through erythromycin ribosomal methyltransferase (erm) genes that modify the binding site for macrolides. It has been known for some time that M fortuitum has a gene coding for erm 39.[26] Induction of this gene is consistent with the trailing endpoints commonly seen during susceptibility testing of M fortuitum isolates against macrolides. M abscessus also possesses a novel erm (41) gene that confers inducible macrolide resistance.[27] This results in "susceptibility" noted at day 3 of incubation and resistance after a maximum incubation period of 14 days. Importantly, M massiliense has a dysfunctional erm gene. The drug resistance profile of 202 M abscessus isolates reported only 16% were susceptible to clarithromycin, 24% were found to be resistant, and 59% noted inducible resistance to clarithromycin.[28] In fact, the erm (41) deletion tends to be species specific (for M massiliense) and perhaps can give a preliminary identification of this species as well as macrolide susceptibility indications quicker than the 14-day extended incubation required for full phenotypic characterization. However, this strain identification target will certainly evolve as larger strain collections from diverse geographic areas are studied.

Choi and colleagues[29] examined the differential effects of clarithromycin and azithromycin induction of the erm (41) in M abscessus and M massiliense isolates. Induction of macrolide resistance was observed in all M abscessus isolates and was significantly greater after exposure to clarithromycin than azithromycin. Clarithromycin induced far greater erm (41) mRNA levels in M abscessus than did azithromycin. None of the M massiliense isolates demonstrated inducible resistance to the macrolides. The drugs were also tested in a murine bone marrow–derived macrophage system, as well as a murine lung infection model. Both macrolides had activity against the

M abscessus, but azithromycin reduced the colony-forming counts significantly more than clarithromycin. Both macrolides were equally effective in the murine models infected with *M massiliense*. This work supports accurate subspeciation of the *M abscessus* complex, because it has clinical implications for the choice of drug therapy. It remains important to understand the mechanisms of resistance to these first-line antibiotics in RGM, because neither clarithromycin nor azithromycin have demonstrated superior treatment efficacy for these infections in humans.[30] To date, there have been no randomized, controlled trials to answer this question.

TREATMENT RECOMMENDATIONS

The diagnosis of pulmonary RGM infection is based on the American Thoracic Society (ATS)/Infectious Diseases Society of America (IDSA) criteria.[1] Treatment for the RGM pulmonary infections is an arduous task for both the patient and the clinician. The multiple medications required, overlapping drug toxicities, long duration of therapy, and discouraging cure rates are analogous to the treatment of multidrug-resistant tuberculosis. For this reason, some patients with minimal symptoms and/or minimal radiographic disease may be better served to follow with watchful waiting before launching into a course of therapy. If therapy is chosen, the clinician and the patient need to determine the goals of therapy, such as symptom improvement, radiographic improvement, or an attempt at cure. The goal of curative therapy is 12 months of culture negativity. Therefore, frequent sputum sampling (every 1–2 months) needs to occur to document when a patient's sputum culture converts to negative.

Treatment for *M abscessus* complex should include 1 to 2 parental agents combined with an oral macrolide in macrolide-susceptible isolates. It is unclear whether the addition of a macrolide offers any clinical benefit in macrolide-resistant disease. Monotherapy with any agent should be avoided, because this may lead to resistance. The most active parenteral agents include amikacin, cefoxitin, imipenem, and tigecycline. Amikacin is recommended to be dosed at 10 to 15 mg/kg per day. In patients with compromised renal function or in whom a long duration of therapy is anticipated, thrice weekly dosing is also used at 15 to 25 mg/kg. Pharmacokinetic testing can help to optimize the dose for each patient based on the MIC for that agent. Cefoxitin should be administered at 200 mg/kg per day with a maximum dose of 12 mg/d in divided doses. Imipenem is typically dosed at 500 to 1000 mg 2 to 4 times

daily. The recommended dosage for tigecycline is 50 mg twice daily, although clinical efficacy has been noted with 50 mg dosed once daily as well[23] in the treatment of mycobacterial infections. Multiple daily doses of any parenteral agent are difficult to administer for outpatients who need to transport themselves to an infusion center for each dose. It is not reasonable to hospitalize patients with a chronic, indolent disease for months at a time. This is a significant obstacle that we face in patients with RGM infections. All patients with *M abscessus* lung disease should be considered for operative resection if they have focal disease, because the outcomes are significantly improved with a combined surgical–medical approach.[2,31] Ideally, operative resection should occur after the infection has been treated with aggressive IV therapy. Surgery should only be performed in an experienced center. Goals of therapy before resection include conversion of sputum smear to negative and optimization of nutritional status. After parenteral therapy is complete, options for step-down therapy include a macrolide with the additional of an oral antibiotic, such as a fluoroquinolone, linezolid, clofazimine, or inhaled amikacin. With the knowledge that *M abscessus* has very low rates of in vitro activity to the macrolides owing to inducible macrolide resistance,[28] perhaps all patients should transition to a combination of a macrolide plus 2 additional agents with in vitro activity (**Fig. 3**).

Treatment of *M chelonae* pulmonary infection is similar to that of *M abscessus*. This organism has a slightly more favorable drug susceptibility pattern. Tobramycin is more active in vitro than amikacin for *M chelonae*. Imipenem is the preferred second parental option, because all isolates of *M chelonae* are resistant to cefoxitin in vitro.[32–34] Antibiotic choice should be based on in vitro susceptibility with at least 2 active agents. Duration of therapy is similar to that of *M abscessus* complex, with the goal of 12 months of culture negativity.[1]

A diagnosis of *M fortuitum* pulmonary infection should provoke a thorough investigation for an aspiration syndrome owing to either defects in the swallowing mechanism or gastroesophageal reflux with aspiration.[2] Fortunately, *M fortuitum* isolates are usually susceptible to multiple oral antimicrobial agents, including the fluoroquinolones, doxycycline, and minocycline, and sulfonamides.[33,35] *M fortuitum* is known to possess an *erm* gene conferring inducible macrolide resistance[26]; therefore macrolides should be used with caution. The ATS/IDSA guidelines recommend treatment of pulmonary disease with at least 2 active agents for 12 months of culture negativity.[1]

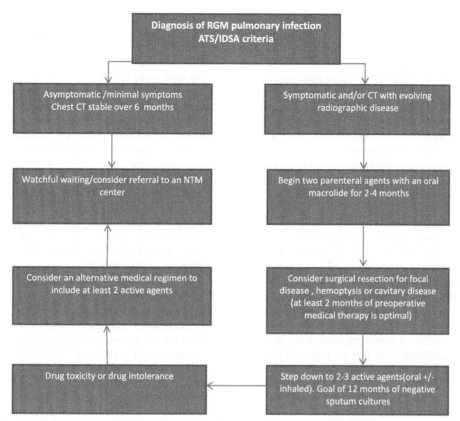

Fig. 3. Algorithm for the management of RGM pulmonary infections. ATS, American Thoracic Society; CT, computed tomography; IDSA, Infectious Diseases Society of America; NTM, nontuberculous mycobacteria; RGM, rapidly growing mycobacteria.

OUTCOMES WITH TREATMENT

In 1993, Griffith and colleagues[2] published their dismal experience in 120 patients with *M abscessus* pulmonary disease. Patients were followed for an average of nearly 5 years and received combination antibiotic therapy including amikacin, cefoxitin, and erythromycin or sulfonamides. Only 10 patients (8%) were able to be cured, 7 of the 10 received IV antibiotics followed by surgical lung resection. Of 120 patients, 18 (15%) died as a result of their chronic lung disease. With this experience, we have historically considered *M abscessus* pulmonary disease a chronic, incurable infection.

It was 16 years before another large series was published. The authors from Samsung Medical Center in Korea published a retrospective analysis of 65 patients who received standardized treatment for *M abscessus* pulmonary disease.[13] All patients received oral clarithromycin, ciprofloxacin, doxycycline, and an initial 4 weeks of IV amikacin in addition to either IV cefoxitin or IV imipenem. Sputum conversion and maintenance of negative cultures for 1 year were noted in 58% of patients. Eighty-three percent had symptom improvement and 74% noted radiographic improvement as well. Adjunctive surgical resection was performed in 14 of these patients (22%). Of 65 patients, 41 (63%) were able to complete therapy with 37 of 65 (57%) undergoing 24 or more months of treatment. Treatment success was associated with in vitro response to clarithromycin, with cure rates of 17% in those patients who were resistant to clarithromycin versus 64% cure in those who were susceptible or intermediate to clarithromycin ($P = .007$). These results were a perplexing breath of fresh air for a disease we had all considered largely incurable.

Later in 2011, the same authors detailed the reasons for the difference in outcomes.[36] In fact, more than one half of their patients formerly identified as *M abscessus* were infected with *M massiliense* infection. This is a species closely related to *M abscessus*; however, its clinical relevance is important because it does not have a functional *erm* gene, which results in a more favorable response to the macrolides. The proportion of patients with sputum conversion and maintenance of negative cultures was greater with *M massiliense* infection than *M abscessus* infection (88% vs 25%; *P*<.001). Inducible clarithromycin resistance was noted in all the tested *M abscessus* isolates, but none of the *M massiliense* isolates.

These same authors also presented outcomes in a later analysis with 34 patients who had *M massiliense* and 24 patients with *M abscessus*.[37] Of 58 patients, 34 (59%) were included in the first study as well.[36] They reported culture conversion rates of 100% in the patients with *M massiliense* infection compared with 50% in *M abscessus* infection, with a median time to culture conversion of 10 and 299 days, respectively. Radiographic improvement was seen in 88% of patients with *M massiliense* infection versus 33% of the time in *M abscessus* infection. Interestingly, 15 of 34 patients (44%) with *M massiliense* infection were noted to have cavitary disease and all of these patients showed cavitary contraction on therapy. Therefore, none of these patients were deemed surgical candidates for the purpose of cavitary resection because the cavities responded so well to therapy. Here, we find another clinical pearl and indication for identification to the species level within the *M abscessus* complex.

Jarand and colleagues[31] presented the treatment experience with *M abscessus* pulmonary infection at National Jewish Health in Denver, Colorado. This was a retrospective study of 69 patients who were followed for a mean duration of 34 months. Patients received a mean of 4.6 drugs for a mean of 52 antibiotic months with a median of 6 months of IV antibiotics. Of those patients, 74% received a macrolide and IV amikacin with or without an additional IV agent. Twenty of the 69 (29%) remained culture positive, 16 of the 69 (23%) converted their cultures but later relapsed, and 33 of the 69 (48%) converted their culture and did not relapse. There was a significant difference in cure rates (culture conversion for $\geq$1 year) in those patients who underwent adjunctive surgical resection in addition to medical therapy (57% vs 28%; *P* = .022; **Fig. 4**).

Authors form the Asan Medical Center in South Korea described their experience in treating 41 patients with *M abscessus* pulmonary disease with parenteral agents.[38] They retrospectively compared 17 patients who were prescribed a macrolide and 1 parenteral (amikacin) agent with 24 patients who received a macrolide and 2 parenteral agents (amikacin and cefoxitin or imipenem). The median duration of parenteral and total antibiotic therapy was 230 and 511 days, respectively.

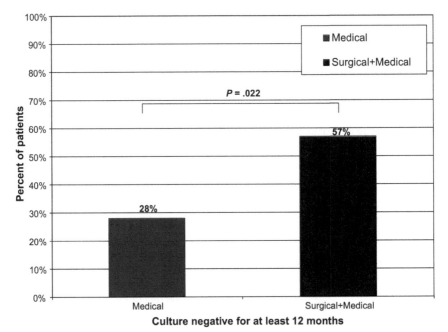

Fig. 4. Microbiologic outcomes in patients receiving medical therapy versus combined medical and surgical therapy for *M abscessus* pulmonary disease. (*Data from* Jarand J, Levin A, Zhang L, et al. Clinical and microbiologic outcomes in patients receiving treatment for Mycobacterium abscessus pulmonary disease. Clin Infect Dis 2011;52(5):565–71.)

Cultures converted to negative in 33 of 41 patients (80.5%) at a median of 151 days. During follow-up, 4 of those 41 patients experienced relapse. This treatment success rate of 70.7% is similar to the outcome originally reported from the Samsung Medical Center in Korea.[13] The authors in this study did not differentiate between M abscessus and M massiliense, which likely contributed to the higher rates of treatment success. Another possible explanation for the higher success rate includes the long duration of IV agents. The imipenem or cefoxitin was prescribed for 2 to 4 months, but the amikacin was administered for a median of 7.6 months. There were no differences in treatment success or relapse rates between the 2 different groups, although the sample sizes were small.

ADVERSE REACTIONS

Medication adverse effects are common in the treatment of nontuberculous mycobacterial infections. Investigators from Ontario noted that patients required a dose reduction or discontinuation of the drug between 18% and 50% of the time for the commonly prescribed antibiotics (ethambutol, rifampin, clarithromycin, or azithromycin).[39] When using medications for the treatment of M abscessus (amikacin, ciprofloxacin, clofazimine, moxifloxacin, cefoxitin, imipenem, or linezolid), the frequency of interruptions owing to side effects was greatly variable (0%–100%).

The M abscessus treatment experience from National Jewish noted that at least 1 drug was stopped because of adverse effects or toxicity in 65% of patients.[31] Cefoxitin and amikacin were most likely to cause adverse effects. Of the patients who received amikacin, 35% developed 1 or more adverse effect, including tinnitus, hearing loss, or vestibular dysfunction. Of 69 patients, 49 (71%) received IV amikacin for at least 1 month; the median number of months of IV amikacin use in this study was 3. Rash was the most common toxicity seen in patients receiving cefoxitin therapy.

In a study from Korea, high rates of cefoxitin toxicity were seen with doses of 200 mg/kg per day.[13] Of 65 patients, 39 (60%) discontinued cefoxitin owing to leukopenia (51%), thrombocytopenia (6%), or transaminitis (15%). No amikacin toxicity was reported with the use of 15 mg/kg per day in 2 divided doses for 4 weeks. Gastrointestinal side effects with the oral agents (clarithromycin, ciprofloxacin, and doxycycline) were seen in 22% of patients.

In a subsequent study from Korea, adverse drug reactions developed in 43.9% of patients in the treatment of M abscessus lung disease.[38] Drug-induced liver injury was seen most often (17%). Leukopenia was seen in 5% of patients. When either of these events occurred, the patient was usually switched from cefoxitin to imipenem and the adverse reaction resolved. Ten percent of patients developed tinnitus or hearing difficulties, 12% had gastrointestinal symptoms, 7.3% noted a rash, and 7.3% had a drug fever.

ADJUNCTIVE SURGICAL RESECTION

We have presented data noting the poor clinical outcomes when medical therapy is used alone. There are several reports now available detailing the surgical outcomes in patients with RGM infections.[31,40–42]

A retrospective study from Korea included 23 patients who underwent pulmonary resection for refractory NTM infection.[42] Only 12 patients had M abscessus infection. The other patients had Mycobacterium avium complex (MAC) or M xenopi infection. The indications for surgery included failure of medical treatment, cavitary lesions, and massive hemoptysis. The median duration of therapy preoperatively was 7.5 months. Of 23 patients, 21 (91%) were able to convert their sputum with surgical therapy and remained negative during the follow-up period. Postoperative complications were high occurring in 35% of patients. There was 1 late postoperative death owing to a bronchopleural fistula 47 days after a completion pneumonectomy.

Another retrospective study from a different group in Korea reported 13 patients who went to surgery for M abscessus pulmonary disease.[38] Only 10 of the 13 patients were able to complete their medical therapy. Six of the 13 patients (46%) were classified as having treatment success. Most of the procedures were through an open thoracotomy (11 of 13; 85%); only 2 had video-assisted thoracoscopic surgery. Postoperative complications occurred in 4 of the 13 patients (30.8%), including postoperative pneumonia (n = 2), bronchopleural fistula (n = 1), and wound dehiscence (n = 1).

The University of Colorado cardiothoracic group has published much lower rates of postoperative complications.[40] They had 134 patients who underwent 172 operations for NTM infection. The vast majority of these operations were through a video-assisted thoracoscopic approach; only 5 cases were converted to an open procedure. Of these 134 patients, 28 (21%) either had primary infection with M abscessus or coinfection with MAC and M abscessus. There was no operative mortality in this series and the postoperative morbidity was quite low (7%). The rate of culture negativity postoperatively was 84% (92/110, with a mean follow-up of 23 months). Eight of these patients eventually had positive cultures again representing relapse or reinfection. Outcomes were not defined between the different types of NTM infection.

A large series of patients with *M abscessus* pulmonary disease who underwent operative resection came from the experience at National Jewish Health.[31] Jarand and colleagues reported outcomes in 69 patients with pulmonary *M abscessus* lung disease. Of the 69 patients, 24 underwent operative resection; of these patients, 15 (65%) were able to convert their cultures to negative and remain negative during the follow-up period (mean duration, 34 months). Postoperative complications were reported in 6 patients (25%).

TREATMENT OF EXTRAPULMONARY RAPIDLY GROWING MYCOBACTERIA INFECTIONS

One of the greatest hurdles in the arena of extrapulmonary mycobacterial infections is the delay in diagnosis. Reasons for this delay include a lack of appreciation for nontuberculous mycobacteria and the indolent nature of these infections. In a large outbreak of postoperative infections, the median time from surgery to the manifestation of clinical symptoms was 31 days (range, 2–187).[43] Occasionally, mycobacteria will be seen in the pathologic examination or cultured from the routine bacterial cultures. Unfortunately, in most cases we do not stumble upon this diagnosis. Acid-fast smears, cultures, and appropriate drug susceptibility testing need to be ordered to reach the diagnosis.

Extrapulmonary infections can involve any organ system. Most commonly, they manifest as skin and soft tissue infection, osteomyelitis, lymphadenitis, or disseminated infection. Often, these organisms are introduced as a result of contaminated medications, medical devices, or injected materials.[43–47] Other outbreaks have been described after acupuncture or pedicures (**Figs. 5** and **6**).[48–50]

In a large, nail salon–associated outbreak of *M fortuitum* furunculosis, we learned that surgical resection was not necessary for cure.[50] Of 61 patients, 48 received antibiotic therapy for a median period of 4 months (range, 1–6). Thirty-three patients received dual therapy and 15 received monotherapy. All treated patients were cured of their infection.

Outbreaks of *M abscessus* complex are not as simple to treat owing to the greater degree of drug resistance. The largest published outbreak

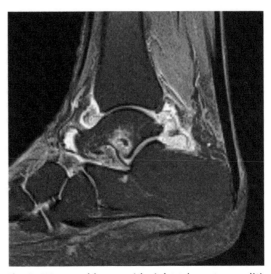

Fig. 5. 55 year old man with right talar osteomyelitis due to *M abscessus*.

to date occurred in Brazil with more than 1000 possible cases of postoperative *M massiliense* infection.[43] Most of the patients were treated with clarithromycin and amikacin or with clarithromycin, amikacin, and a third injectable agent (either imipenem or cefoxitin) with good clinical outcomes. In addition, most of these patients underwent surgical debridement and abscess drainage.

In a series of 15 patients who developed cesarean section surgical site infections with *M abscessus*, most patients (14/15) required surgical debridement with prolonged combination medical therapy.[51] The mean ± standard deviation duration of combined parenteral therapy was 28 ± 8 days; then, all 14 patients received monotherapy with clarithromycin for a mean of 23 ± 13 weeks.

M fortuitum infections are easier to manage than *M abscessus* complex or *M chelonae*. Patients

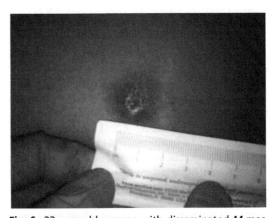

Fig. 6. 23 year old woman with disseminated *M massiliense* infection. Each skin lesion is similar with a raised violaceous appearance. Central umbilication with spontaneous suppuration is noted.

with *M fortuitum* should receive at least 2 active agents for skin and soft tissue infection. Consider parenteral therapy initially for *M fortuitum* osteomyelitis. When managing *M chelonae* or *M abscessus* extrapulmonary infections, more aggressive management is warranted owing to the drug resistance of these organisms. Two to 3 active agents (with parenteral therapy initially) should be administered.

Surgery is advised in extensive disease, abscess formation, drug resistance, or when drug therapy is difficult. Our experience supports early operative intervention with extrapulmonary RGM infections, excluding *M fortuitum*. In all the RGM infections, removal of foreign material is imperative for cure (ie, catheters, implantable devices). In general, skin and soft tissue infections should be treated for a minimum of 4 months and for at least 6 months if there is bone involvement. Our practice is to continue antibiotic therapy for at least 2 months beyond the resolution of all clinical signs of active infection.

TREATMENT COST

The median medication cost in treating NTM infections is estimated to be $19,876 (range, $398–70,917).[52] In this analysis, the cost varied greatly depending on the infecting organism. Patients with MAC had a median medication cost of $14,730 compared with an overall median cost of $47,240 for those patients with *M abscessus* infection. The average monthly cost for imipenem or cefoxitin in the United States was $3259 to $3403, respectively. The average monthly cost for amikacin is $161 in the United States. This is an underestimate of the total cost of treatment, because this study did not measure the cost of administering IV medications, outpatient visits, or hospitalizations. When compared with other chronic infectious diseases, the authors estimate the cost is similar to treating a patient with human immunodeficiency virus or AIDS.[53,54]

Another estimation of cost was published based on experience in an Ontario health care system.[39] In this retrospective review, the authors analyzed cost for 91 patients with pulmonary NTM disease. The vast majority of patients had MAC infection; only 7% were infected with *M abscessus*. The median monthly cost of a standard first line regimen for MAC was only $245 Canadian dollars compared with $470 US dollars in the study by Ballarino and colleagues. The monthly cost significantly increased if IV therapies were included in the Canadian regimen (median monthly cost CAD 1161).

NEW DRUGS ARE NEEDED

Mycobacterial pathogens are intrinsically resistant to most antibiotics and cause significant morbidity. Although *Mycobacterium tuberculosis* has been the subject of extensive drug discovery efforts, the nontuberculous mycobacteria pose a unique therapeutic challenge. Current treatment options for NTM are limited. There is interest in testing new anti–*M tuberculosis* compounds against NTM and there have even been nascent programs specifically designed to develop and test NTM-specific drugs. Unfortunately, therapeutic agents developed to treat *M tuberculosis* infections often lack activity against NTM and, even when compounds demonstrate good in vitro MICs, there is often an absence of bactericidal activity.[55,56] Thus, new potent treatment options for NTM are still not available. As an example, the US Food and Drug Administration recently approved diarylquinoline antibiotic bedaquiline (BDQ); it is currently in phase III testing in patients with pulmonary multidrug resistant tuberculosis and is approved for this indication based on early priority clearance by the US Food and Drug Administration. Although future human clinical trials may be conducted in NTM disease with BDQ, it remains to be determined whether this agent will be useful. Although BDQ has excellent bacteriostatic in vitro activity against *M avium* and *M abscessus*, it lacks bactericidal activity in vitro and in vivo.[56,57] Drugs with only bacteriostatic activity are not necessarily without utility. It is crucial to rigorously examine the preclinical activity of this and other new drugs before treatment trials in humans. To accomplish this with BDQ and any new agent with promising activity, the preclinical animal models that are still in development need more validation. In addition, there is a need to generate data combining new agents such as BDQ with drugs that are currently used to treat *M abscessus*, namely, clarithromycin, cefoxitin, imipenem, tigecycline, and amikacin.

To do this will require a dedicated effort and funding to test new antibiotics and agents with host immunomodulatory properties in relevant in vivo models for NTM. Historically, antimycobacterial drug discovery and preclinical testing efforts have focused almost exclusively on *M tuberculosis*, with virtually no concerted effort going toward extended spectrum agents that cover NTM. However, with the increased funding for in vitro and in vivo NTM drug testing contracts under the National Institutes of Health (www.niaid.nih.gov/labsandresources/resources/dmid/Pages/default.aspx), this is fortunately changing. As part of the whole preclinical pathway, robust acute and chronic infection models for the most highly relevant NTM pathogens are needed.

PRECLINICAL MODELS BEING DEVELOPED FOR TESTING NEW AGENTS

Successful models for in vivo testing in an RGM NTM infection model are a critical part of new drug development. A number of murine models of RGM infection have been described, including SCID,[58] nude,[57,59] granulocyte macrophage colony stimulating factor–gene disrupted mice, cystic fibrosis mouse models,[59] and gamma interferon knockout mice.[60] More recently, alternative models including a fruit fly model that does not display typical mammalian pathologic features has proved useful for studying NTM active compounds.[61] It has been challenging to find a productive model of infection with lesions that resemble those of the human lung disease. The granulocyte macrophage colony stimulating factor knockout mouse model has demonstrated chronic infection and histopathologic evidence of pneumonia and bronchiectasis.[62] The establishment of a persistent infection would allow assessments of activities of agents in acute infections as well as to identify those compounds with activity in chronic, well-established infection with lesions resembling human pathology. Taking the lead from lessons learned with *M tuberculosis* preclinical models,[63] a variety of carefully planned and executed preclinical models will need to be employed that reflect and recapitulate the heterogeneity of RGM human infections and are reproducible. A variety of animal models may need to be employed to capture the heterogenous nature of human diseases (chronic pulmonary infections and disseminated disease, as well as cutaneous manifestations). Although challenging to treat with current antimicrobial regimens, interest in RGM-specific drug discovery platforms and new animal models as well as the first ever multicenter, randomized, controlled trial of a novel formulation of inhaled amikacin (Arykase)[64] offer novel and brighter opportunities for treatment of patients infected with these important pathogens.

ACKNOWLEDGMENTS

The authors thank Koen Andries for helpful discussions.

REFERENCES

1. Griffith DE, Aksamit T, Brown-Elliott BA, et al. An official ATS/IDSA statement: diagnosis, treatment, and prevention of nontuberculous mycobacterial diseases. Am J Respir Crit Care Med 2007;175(4): 367–416.
2. Griffith DE, Girard WM, Wallace RJ Jr. Clinical features of pulmonary disease caused by rapidly growing mycobacteria. An analysis of 154 patients. Am Rev Respir Dis 1993;147(5):1271–8.
3. Daley CL, Griffith DE. Pulmonary disease caused by rapidly growing mycobacteria. Clin Chest Med 2002;23(3):623–32, vii.
4. Macheras E, Konjek J, Roux AL, et al. Multilocus sequence typing scheme for the Mycobacterium abscessus complex. Res Microbiol 2014;165(2):82–90.
5. Sassi M, Drancourt M. Genome analysis reveals three genomospecies in Mycobacterium abscessus. BMC Genomics 2014;15:359.
6. Bryant JM, Grogono DM, Greaves D, et al. Whole-genome sequencing to identify transmission of Mycobacterium abscessus between patients with cystic fibrosis: a retrospective cohort study. Lancet 2013;381(9877):1551–60.
7. Howard ST. Recent progress towards understanding genetic variation in the Mycobacterium abscessus complex. Tuberculosis 2013;93(Suppl):S15–20.
8. Tettelin H, Davidson RM, Agrawal S, et al. High-level relatedness among Mycobacterium abscessus subsp. massiliense strains from widely separated outbreaks. Emerg Infect Dis 2014;20(3):364–71.
9. Aitken ML, Limaye A, Pottinger P, et al. Respiratory outbreak of Mycobacterium abscessus subspecies massiliense in a lung transplant and cystic fibrosis center. Am J Respir Crit Care Med 2012;185(2): 231–2.
10. Bottger EC. Transmission of M abscessus in patients with cystic fibrosis. Lancet 2013;382(9891):503–4.
11. Shin SJ, Choi GE, Cho SN, et al. Mycobacterial genotypes are associated with clinical manifestation and progression of lung disease caused by Mycobacterium abscessus and Mycobacterium massiliense. Clin Infect Dis 2013;57(1):32–9.
12. Harada T, Akiyama Y, Kurashima A, et al. Clinical and microbiological differences between Mycobacterium abscessus and Mycobacterium massiliense lung diseases. J Clin Microbiol 2012;50(11):3556–61.
13. Jeon K, Kwon OJ, Lee NY, et al. Antibiotic treatment of Mycobacterium abscessus lung disease: a retrospective analysis of 65 patients. Am J Respir Crit Care Med 2009;180(9):896–902.
14. Park S, Kim S, Park EM, et al. In vitro antimicrobial susceptibility of Mycobacterium abscessus in Korea. J Korean Med Sci 2008;23(1):49–52.
15. Zhuo FL, Sun ZG, Li CY, et al. Clinical isolates of Mycobacterium abscessus in Guangzhou area most possibly from the environmental infection showed variable susceptibility. Chin Med J 2013; 126(10):1878–83.
16. Huang YC, Liu MF, Shen GH, et al. Clinical outcome of Mycobacterium abscessus infection and

antimicrobial susceptibility testing. J Microbiol Immunol Infect 2010;43(5):401–6.

17. Reddy VM, O'Sullivan JF, Gangadharam PR. Antimycobacterial activities of riminophenazines. J Antimicrob Chemother 1999;43(5):615–23.

18. Shen GH, Wu BD, Hu ST, et al. High efficacy of clofazimine and its synergistic effect with amikacin against rapidly growing mycobacteria. Int J Antimicrob Agents 2010;35(4):400–4.

19. van Ingen J, Totten SE, Helstrom NK, et al. In vitro synergy between clofazimine and amikacin in treatment of nontuberculous mycobacterial disease. Antimicrob Agents Chemother 2012;56(12):6324–7.

20. Wallace RJ Jr, Brown-Elliott BA, Crist CJ, et al. Comparison of the in vitro activity of the glycylcycline tigecycline (formerly GAR-936) with those of tetracycline, minocycline, and doxycycline against isolates of nontuberculous mycobacteria. Antimicrob Agents Chemother 2002;46(10):3164–7.

21. Garrison AP, Morris MI, Doblecki Lewis S, et al. Mycobacterium abscessus infection in solid organ transplant recipients: report of three cases and review of the literature. Transpl Infect Dis 2009;11(6):541–8.

22. Peres E, Khaled Y, Krijanovski OI, et al. Mycobacterium chelonae necrotizing pneumonia after allogeneic hematopoietic stem cell transplant: report of clinical response to treatment with tigecycline. Transpl Infect Dis 2009;11(1):57–63.

23. Wallace RJ Jr, Dukart G, Brown-Elliott BA, et al. Clinical experience in 52 patients with tigecycline-containing regimens for salvage treatment of Mycobacterium abscessus and Mycobacterium chelonae infections. J Antimicrob Chemother 2014;69(7):1945–53.

24. Greendyke R, Byrd TF. Differential antibiotic susceptibility of Mycobacterium abscessus variants in biofilms and macrophages compared to that of planktonic bacteria. Antimicrob Agents Chemother 2008;52(6):2019–26.

25. Wallace RJ Jr, Meier A, Brown BA, et al. Genetic basis for clarithromycin resistance among isolates of Mycobacterium chelonae and Mycobacterium abscessus. Antimicrob Agents Chemother 1996;40(7):1676–81.

26. Nash KA, Zhang Y, Brown-Elliott BA, et al. Molecular basis of intrinsic macrolide resistance in clinical isolates of Mycobacterium fortuitum. J Antimicrob Chemother 2005;55(2):170–7.

27. Nash KA, Brown-Elliott BA, Wallace RJ Jr. A novel gene, erm(41), confers inducible macrolide resistance to clinical isolates of Mycobacterium abscessus but is absent from Mycobacterium chelonae. Antimicrob Agents Chemother 2009;53(4):1367–76.

28. Lee SH, Yoo HK, Kim SH, et al. The drug resistance profile of Mycobacterium abscessus group strains from Korea. Ann Lab Med 2014;34(1):31–7.

29. Choi GE, Shin SJ, Won CJ, et al. Macrolide treatment for Mycobacterium abscessus and Mycobacterium massiliense infection and inducible resistance. Am J Respir Crit Care Med 2012;186(9):917–25.

30. Maurer FP, Castelberg C, Quiblier C, et al. Erm(41)-dependent inducible resistance to azithromycin and clarithromycin in clinical isolates of Mycobacterium abscessus. J Antimicrob Chemother 2014;69(6):1559–63.

31. Jarand J, Levin A, Zhang L, et al. Clinical and microbiologic outcomes in patients receiving treatment for Mycobacterium abscessus pulmonary disease. Clin Infect Dis 2011;52(5):565–71.

32. Broda A, Jebbari H, Beaton K, et al. Comparative drug resistance of Mycobacterium abscessus and M. chelonae isolates from patients with and without cystic fibrosis in the United Kingdom. J Clin Microbiol 2013;51(1):217–23.

33. Swenson JM, Wallace RJ Jr, Silcox VA, et al. Antimicrobial susceptibility of five subgroups of Mycobacterium fortuitum and Mycobacterium chelonae. Antimicrob Agents Chemother 1985;28(6):807–11.

34. Brown BA, Wallace RJ Jr, Onyi GO, et al. Activities of four macrolides, including clarithromycin, against Mycobacterium fortuitum, Mycobacterium chelonae, and M. chelonae-like organisms. Antimicrob Agents Chemother 1992;36(1):180–4.

35. Wallace RJ Jr, Steele LC, Forrester GD, et al. Susceptibilities of Mycobacterium fortuitum biovariant fortuitum and the unnamed third biovariant complex to heavy-metal salts. Antimicrob Agents Chemother 1984;26(4):594–6.

36. Koh WJ, Jeon K, Lee NY, et al. Clinical significance of differentiation of Mycobacterium massiliense from Mycobacterium abscessus. Am J Respir Crit Care Med 2011;183(3):405–10.

37. Kim HS, Lee KS, Koh WJ, et al. Serial CT findings of Mycobacterium massiliense pulmonary disease compared with Mycobacterium abscessus disease after treatment with antibiotic therapy. Radiology 2012;263(1):260–70.

38. Lyu J, Jang HJ, Song JW, et al. Outcomes in patients with Mycobacterium abscessus pulmonary disease treated with long-term injectable drugs. Respir Med 2011;105(5):781–7.

39. Leber A, Marras TK. The cost of medical management of pulmonary nontuberculous mycobacterial disease in Ontario, Canada. Eur Respir J 2011;37(5):1158–65.

40. Yu JA, Pomerantz M, Bishop A, et al. Lady Windermere revisited: treatment with thoracoscopic lobectomy/segmentectomy for right middle lobe and lingular bronchiectasis associated with non-tuberculous mycobacterial disease. Eur J Cardiothorac Surg 2011;40(3):671–5.

41. Sugino K, Kobayashi M, Iwata M, et al. Successful treatment with pneumonectomy for pulmonary

Mycobacterium abscessus infection. Intern Med 2009;48(6):459–63.

42. Koh WJ, Kim YH, Kwon OJ, et al. Surgical treatment of pulmonary diseases due to nontuberculous mycobacteria. J Korean Med Sci 2008;23(3):397–401.

43. Duarte RS, Lourenco MC, Fonseca Lde S, et al. Epidemic of postsurgical infections caused by Mycobacterium massiliense. J Clin Microbiol 2009; 47(7):2149–55.

44. Furuya EY, Paez A, Srinivasan A, et al. Outbreak of Mycobacterium abscessus wound infections among "ipotourists" from the United States who underwent abdominoplasty in the Dominican Republic. Clin Infect Dis 2008;46(8):1181–8.

45. Tiwari TS, Ray B, Jost KC Jr, et al. Forty years of disinfectant failure: outbreak of postinjection Mycobacterium abscessus infection caused by contamination of benzalkonium chloride. Clin Infect Dis 2003;36(8):954–62.

46. Munayco CV, Grijalva CG, Culqui DR, et al. Outbreak of persistent cutaneous abscesses due to Mycobacterium chelonae after mesotherapy sessions, Lima, Peru. Rev Saude Publica 2008;42(1):146–9.

47. Kennedy BS, Bedard B, Younge M, et al. Outbreak of Mycobacterium chelonae infection associated with tattoo ink. N Engl J Med 2012;367(11):1020–4.

48. Song JY, Sohn JW, Jeong HW, et al. An outbreak of post-acupuncture cutaneous infection due to Mycobacterium abscessus. BMC Infect Dis 2006;6:6.

49. Sniezek PJ, Graham BS, Busch HB, et al. Rapidly growing mycobacterial infections after pedicures. Arch Dermatol 2003;139(5):629–34.

50. Winthrop KL, Albridge K, South D, et al. The clinical management and outcome of nail salon-acquired Mycobacterium fortuitum skin infection. Clin Infect Dis 2004;38(1):38–44.

51. Tsao SM, Liu KS, Liao HH, et al. The clinical management of cesarean section-acquired Mycobacterium abscessus surgical site infections. J Infect Dev Ctries 2014;8(2):184–92.

52. Ballarino GJ, Olivier KN, Claypool RJ, et al. Pulmonary nontuberculous mycobacterial infections: antibiotic treatment and associated costs. Respir Med 2009;103(10):1448–55.

53. Schackman BR, Gebo KA, Walensky RP, et al. The lifetime cost of current human immunodeficiency virus care in the United States. Med Care 2006;44(11):990–7.

54. Hutchinson AB, Farnham PG, Dean HD, et al. The economic burden of HIV in the United States in the era of highly active antiretroviral therapy: evidence of continuing racial and ethnic differences. J Acquir Immune Defic Syndr 2006;43(4):451–7.

55. Maurer FP, Bruderer VL, Ritter C, et al. Lack of antimicrobial bactericidal activity in Mycobacterium abscessus. Antimicrob Agents Chemother 2014;58(7): 3828–36.

56. Lounis N, Gevers T, Van den Berg J, et al. ATP synthase inhibition of Mycobacterium avium is not bactericidal. Antimicrob Agents Chemother 2009; 53(11):4927–9.

57. Lerat I, Cambau E, Roth Dit Bettoni R, et al. In vivo evaluation of antibiotic activity against Mycobacterium abscessus. J Infect Dis 2014;209(6):905–12.

58. Howard ST, Rhoades E, Recht J, et al. Spontaneous reversion of Mycobacterium abscessus from a smooth to a rough morphotype is associated with reduced expression of glycopeptidolipid and reacquisition of an invasive phenotype. Microbiology 2006;152(Pt 6):1581–90.

59. Orme IM, Ordway DJ. The host response to nontuberculous mycobacterial infections of current clinical importance. Infect Immun 2014;82:3516–22.

60. Ordway D, Henao-Tamayo M, Smith E, et al. Animal model of Mycobacterium abscessus lung infection. J Leukoc Biol 2008;83(6):1502–11.

61. Oh CT, Moon C, Park OK, et al. Novel drug combination for Mycobacterium abscessus disease therapy identified in a Drosophila infection model. J Antimicrob Chemother 2014;69(6):1599–607.

62. De Groote MA, Johnson L, Podell B, et al. GM-CSF knockout mice for preclinical testing of agents with antimicrobial activity against Mycobacterium abscessus. J Antimicrob Chemother 2014;69(4):1057–64.

63. Franzblau SG, DeGroote MA, Cho SH, et al. Comprehensive analysis of methods used for the evaluation of compounds against Mycobacterium tuberculosis. Tuberculosis 2012;92(6):453–88.

64. Olivier KN, Gupta R, Daley CL, et al. A randomized, double-blind, placebo-controlled study of liposomal amikacin for inhalation (Arikace®) in patients with recalcitrant nontuberculous mycobacterial lung disease [Publication Number: A4126]. Presented to the American Thoracic Society. San Diego, May 2014.

Treatment of Slowly Growing Mycobacteria

Julie V. Philley, MD*, David E. Griffith, MD

KEYWORDS

- Nontuberculous mycobacteria • Mycobacterial disease • MAC • *Mycobacterium avium* complex
- *M avium* • Bronchiectasis • NTM • Slow-growing mycobacteria

KEY POINTS

- The treatment of slow-growing mycobacteria requires a multidrug regimen and a long course of therapy, typically 12 to 18 months.
- The only drugs for which in vitro susceptibilities correlate with an in vivo response in MAC lung disease are macrolides and amikacin.
- Patients with macrolide-resistant MAC and patients who do not respond to standard therapy require early referral and treatment at a specialized center.
- Inhaled amikacin may provide an adjunct therapy for the treatment of MAC lung disease, but adequate companion drugs are necessary to prevent the emergence of amikacin resistance.

INTRODUCTION

Historically, mycobacteria that form colonies visible to the naked eye in more than 7 days on subculture media are termed slow growers. Slowly growing nontuberculous mycobacterial (NTM) species include *Mycobacterium avium* complex (MAC) (*M intracellulare, M avium, M chimaera*), *M kansasii, M haemophilum, M marinum,* and *M ulcerans.* Less commonly encountered pathogens in the United States include *M scrofulaceum, M malmoense, M simiae, M szulgai, M terrae complex,* and *M xenopi,* although the latter is a significant source of lung disease in Canada, Northern Europe, and other parts of the world. Slowly growing NTM species were the first NTM to be recognized as causing chronic lung disease.

PATIENT EVALUATION OVERVIEW

Slowly growing NTM lung disease, especially caused by MAC, is broadly associated with 2 distinct radiographic forms of disease. The first to be described involves upper lobe fibrocavitary densities resembling pulmonary tuberculosis and occurs primarily in men with underlying obstructive lung disease (**Fig. 1**A). The second radiographic manifestation involves nodules and bronchiectasis and occurs primarily in women without underlying pulmonary disease other than bronchiectasis and in the United States is the most common presentation of the most common slowly growing NTM pathogen, MAC (see **Fig. 1**B). Although MAC is the best described NTM pathogen with this radiographic dichotomy, it has also been described with most other slowly growing NTM pathogens.[1]

Kim and colleagues[2] from the National Institutes of Health (NIH) reported 63 patients (95% female) with NTM lung disease and a characteristic body habitus including lower body weight and significantly greater height than matched controls. These patients also had higher rates of scoliosis (51%), pectus excavatum (11%), and mitral valve prolapse (9%) compared with matched controls. No cytokine pathway abnormalities or cell-mediated dysfunction were found in these patients. In a recent similar report, investigators

Disclosure: Dr. Philley served on an advisory board for Insmed Pharmaceuticals in 2014.
Department of Medicine, University of Texas Health Science Center, 11037 US Highway 271, Tyler, TX 75708, USA
* Corresponding author. 11937 US Highway 271, Tyler, TX 75708.
E-mail address: Julie.philley@uthct.edu

Clin Chest Med 36 (2015) 79–90
http://dx.doi.org/10.1016/j.ccm.2014.10.005
0272-5231/15/$ – see front matter © 2015 Elsevier Inc. All rights reserved.

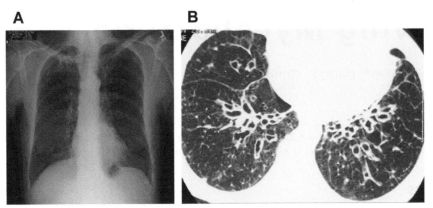

Fig. 1. (*A*) A 79-year-old man with greater than 100 pack year history of cigarette smoking and severe emphysema, who presented with worsening cough, fatigue, and weight loss. Posteroanterior chest radiograph shows right upper lobe cavitary lesion, with dense surrounding inflammatory changes. Sputum cultures were positive for *M xenopi* on multiple specimens. The patient was successfully treated with azithromycin, ethambutol, and rifampin. (*B*) A 68-year-old woman with bronchiectasis by chest computed tomography.

from National Jewish Health[3] again noted the characteristic body habitus of female patients with MAC lung disease but, in contrast to the NIH study, found decreased cytokine (interferon γ and interleukin 10) response of stimulated peripheral blood monocytes from patients with MAC compared with controls.

The NIH study also found a higher incidence of cystic fibrosis (CF) transmembrane conductance regulator (CFTR) gene mutations (36%) compared with a matched control population, although there was no consistent correlation between sweat chloride concentrations and CFTR variants. It has also been noted in Japan[4] that patients with pulmonary NTM disease have CFTR gene mutations more frequently than in the general population. In a recent study,[5] patients heterozygous for CFTR mutations were found to have abnormal nasal potential differences compared with controls, suggesting a subtle mucosal ion transport abnormality and a possible pathophysiologic pathway for developing bronchiectasis. However, there is no clear connection between single CFTR mutations and the characteristic body habitus described earlier or a clearly delineated mechanism through which a single CFTR mutation might cause bronchiectasis.

The consensus among most NTM lung disease experts is that bronchiectasis precedes and predisposes to NTM infection similar to what is observed in patients with CF.[6,7] However, some patients with NTM lung disease associated with nodules and bronchiectasis have nodular infiltrate, which may precede the development of cylindrical bronchiectasis. For these patients, therefore, NTM infection might be the cause of their bronchiectasis. In the absence of early and sensitive measures to detect bronchiectasis or an animal model of chronic NTM lung disease, this chicken and egg question is impossible to answer for many patients. Likely, there are many phenotypic pathways to the development of bronchiectasis with or without NTM lung disease. From a practical standpoint, patients with known bronchiectasis for any reason should be screened for NTM infection and should be considered for evaluation of genetic or hereditary causes of bronchiectasis.

Although the current research and public health emphasis in the United States is on NTM lung disease associated with nodules and bronchiectasis, it is important not to forget the fibrocavitary form of slowly growing NTM lung disease, which more closely resembles tuberculosis radiographically and clinically. *M avium* complex lung infection was initially recognized with this radiographic manifestation, and in some areas in the United States, it still accounts for much of the observed MAC lung disease. Other slowly growing respiratory NTM pathogens such as *M xenopi*, *M kansasii*, *M szulagi*, and *M malmoense* present more frequently with cavitary lung abnormalities than with nodules and bronchiectasis. In contrast to the United States, in some parts of the world, especially Western Europe, fibrocavitary NTM disease is more common overall than disease associated with nodules and bronchiectasis.[8,9] An important predisposing association for the development of cavitary NTM lung disease seems to be cigarette smoking.[10,11] In that regard, cavitary NTM lung disease is pathophysiologically distinct from nodular/bronchiectasic disease and should probably be considered another in a long list of cigarette smoking–related diseases. Although there are important pathophysiologic differences, both disease presentations seem to require the presence of an underlying airway abnormality that promotes or facilitates NTM infection.

Ito and colleagues[11] described predictors of 5-year mortality in patients with MAC lung disease. After adjusting for multiple cofounders, the presence of cavitary disease was associated with a higher mortality than disease associated with nodules and bronchiectasis, a result confirmed by others.[12,13] Reports of other slowly growing NTM pathogens such as M xenopi also show increased mortality with cavitary lung disease.[8] Although the decision to treat patients with the nodular/bronchiectatic form of NTM lung disease should be based on potential risks and benefits of therapy for individual patients, patients with cavitary lesions require immediate treatment to minimize disease morbidity and mortality.

PHARMACOLOGIC TREATMENT OPTIONS
Mycobacterium avium Complex

There are multiple impediments to successful MAC lung disease therapy that are pertinent, at least to some degree, to other slowly growing NTM pathogens. It is all too familiar to clinicians that treatment outcomes for MAC lung disease are in general less successful than treatment outcomes for tuberculosis. The explanation(s) for this observation are likely multiple and not readily apparent but are the subject of intense investigation.

Perhaps the most frustrating aspect of NTM lung disease management is the observation that in vitro susceptibility testing may not be a guide for effective in vivo response to antibiotics, as it is in the therapy for tuberculosis.[14] The most clinically important example of this phenomenon is MAC, in which, until recently (see later discussion), there was evidence only to support a correlation between in vitro macrolide susceptibility and in vivo clinical response. Both the Clinical and Laboratory Standard Institute (CLSI) and the American Thoracic Society (ATS) recommend that new MAC isolates should be tested in vitro only for susceptibility to macrolides.[14,15] Understandably, clinicians still cling to in vitro susceptibility reports for MAC isolates that list multiple agents as either susceptible or resistant based on in vitro minimum inhibitory concentrations (MICs), even although those MICs have not been shown to correlate with in vivo response to the antibiotics tested. One of several examples of this phenomenon was reported from Japan by Kobashi and colleagues[16] in a study showing a lack of correlation between in vitro susceptibility for MAC and in vivo response to rifampin, ethambutol, and streptomycin.[16] This paradoxic observation has been repeatedly confirmed and attributed to innate resistance, which refers to multiple mycobacterial defenses against antimicrobial agents that may not be reflected by in vitro MICs.[17–20] The discovery of the inducible macrolide resistance or erm gene for M abscessus is an example of 1 such innate resistance mechanism.[8] Clearly, there is a need for better understanding of these innate resistance mechanisms, which, it is hoped, will lead to more effective treatment strategies.

In the context of innate antibiotic resistance, the most obvious explanation for the suboptimal response to antimicrobial agents is the poor antimycobacterial activity of medication choices. In addition to poor antimycobacterial activity, a recent study has shown that recommended macrolide-based treatment regimens for MAC are associated with significant pharmacologic interactions, resulting in low plasma concentrations of all drugs, including macrolides.[21,22] Targeted levels for pharmacodynamic indices for essentially all drugs commonly used in MAC treatment regimens were seldom met. This study did not provide correlation between the suboptimal pharmacodynamic indices with patient outcome. Improvement in the pharmacodynamic parameters would almost certainly entail increased dosages of the MAC medications, which would be a formidable obstacle to overcome for many patients on MAC therapy. MAC medications are weak antimicrobials, which because of drug-drug interactions are usually associated with suboptimal pharmacodynamic indices in patients who cannot tolerate higher doses of the medications to alter those suboptimal indices.

Another possible impediment to favorable treatment outcomes is the lack of adherence by practitioners to published treatment guidelines. In a survey of primarily pulmonary and infectious disease specialists who identified themselves as treating patients with NTM lung disease, fewer than one-third followed published treatment guidelines and as many as 30% prescribed medication regimens that could promote resistance to macrolides.[23] The reasons for the lack of adherence to the published treatment guidelines were not addressed.

A recent study from Ontario[24] that compared practices and perceptions of prognosis for MAC lung disease between experts and nonexperts found less discordance in prescribing practices. Areas of agreement between experts and nonexperts included the first choice of therapy (guideline-directed regimens) and typical duration of treatment. Noted differences were that nonexperts estimated that fewer patients with a positive culture had disease and used suggested guidelines therapy less often in new cases and achieved a slightly lower success rate than with guidelines therapy.

There is clearly a perception, and perhaps rightly, that the published NTM treatment guidelines are inadequate for treating many patients with MAC lung disease. However, recent studies suggest that adherence to these guidelines at least establishes a reasonable baseline for treatment success and that perceived treatment failure may result from circumstances such as microbiological recurrence caused by reinfection that are not necessarily a consequence of a poor or inadequate treatment regimen.[25]

The role of macrolides as the cornerstone of MAC therapy was reinforced by a recently published study[25] evaluating 180 patients with MAC lung disease with nodular bronchiectatic disease who were treated with macrolide-based regimens over an approximately 10-year period. In the study, 84% of patients obtained sputum acid-fast bacilli (AFB) culture conversion with a 3-drug regimen, comprising macrolide, ethambutol, and rifamycin. Most patients did not tolerate daily therapy with this 3-drug regimen but were able to tolerate medication administration 3 times weekly. Microbiological recurrence was common and most frequently caused by new MAC genotypes, which were interpreted as evidence of reinfection rather than as true microbiological relapse. No patient developed macrolide resistance on the 3-drug macrolide-based regimen.

Three-drug macrolide-based therapy with ethambutol and a rifamycin has been recommended as standard MAC therapy based on generally favorable treatment responses over the last approximately 20 years (**Table 1**). The efficacy of 2-drug therapy with macrolide and ethambutol has not been examined rigorously. Miwa and colleagues[26] recently reported a study comparing a 3-drug MAC treatment regimen comprising clarithromycin, ethambutol, and rifampin with a 2-drug regimen comprising only clarithromycin and ethambutol in 119 patients. The rate of sputum culture conversion after 12 months of therapy was 41% with a 3-drug regimen and 55% with a 2-drug regimen. Adverse events leading to discontinuation of treatment occurred in 37% with a 3-drug regimen and 27% in the 2-drug regimen. Macrolide resistance did not occur in either treatment arm. As is the case with the interpretation of many similar uncontrolled studies of NTM therapy, it is still unclear if the 2-drug regimen can be used in place of the standard 3-drug regimen for most patients with MAC lung disease.

Although treatment outcomes for MAC lung disease with standard macrolide-based regimens are generally favorable, better therapeutic regimens with more effective agents are unquestionably needed. The role of inhaled amikacin in a treatment regimen for advanced or recalcitrant NTM lung disease remains uncertain, with few available published data.[27,28] An initial trial in a few patients suggested that inhaled amikacin might be effective, although for almost a decade, there were no corroborating studies. One recent study[28] involved administration of inhaled amikacin to patients with treatment-refractory *M abscessus* and MAC followed for a median of 19 months. Twenty-five percent of these patients had sustained negative AFB cultures while receiving the inhaled amikacin. Patients had a variable symptomatic and objective response to the amikacin, and 35% of patients stopped amikacin because of side effects or adverse events. A multicenter clinical trial investigating the addition of inhaled liposomal amikacin to a stable regimen for recalcitrant MAC and *M abscessus* lung disease was recently completed.[29] In the study, after only 3 months of the inhaled liposomal amikacin preparation, approximately 30% of patients with MAC converted sputum for AFB culture negative after a median of 1 month of therapy. The placebo-controlled and blinded phase of the study was followed by an open-label phase, which was associated with further sputum AFB culture conversion in patients who initially received placebo. Seventy-three percent of patients had side effects or adverse events attributable to the drug, and 16% discontinued the medication because of these side effects or adverse events. In this small and preliminary study, it seems that the liposomal amikacin preparation has the potential to add significantly to the therapy for patients with otherwise treatment-refractory MAC lung disease.

Although fluoroquinolones have been frequently used for MAC lung disease over many years, there has been little evidence to support their use as first-line agents for treating MAC. The use of macrolide and fluoroquinolone without other companion drugs places the patient at risk for development of macrolide-resistant MAC disease. In addition, both drug classes are associated with a prolonged QT interval on an electrocardiogram, which may predispose to cardiac toxicity and excess mortality.[30,31] A recent study[32] evaluated the effect of adding moxifloxacin in 41 patients with MAC lung disease who did not have sputum conversion after at least 6 months of a macrolide-containing regimen. With a median moxifloxacin administration duration of greater than 300 days, the overall treatment success rate was 29%, and the median time to sputum conversion was 91 days. A positive sputum AFB smear at the start of treatment with moxifloxacin-containing

Table 1
Treatment of common slowly growing mycobacteria

NTM	Drug Regimen	Duration of Therapy
M avium complex (MAC)	Nodular/bronchiectasis: Clarithromycin 500 mg by mouth BID or TIW or azithromycin 250 mg by mouth daily or 500–600 mg by mouth TIW plus Ethambutol 15 mg/kg by mouth daily or 25 mg/kg by mouth TIW plus Rifampin 600 mg by mouth daily or TIW or rifabutin 150–300 mg by mouth daily or 300 mg TIW Cavitary: Azithromycin 250–500 mg by mouth daily or clarithromycin 500 mg BID plus Ethambutol 15 mg/kg by mouth daily plus Rifampin 600 mg or rifabutin 150–300 mg by mouth daily plus Streptomycin 5–15 mg/kg IM or IV TIW or amikacin 5–15 mg/kg IV TIW for ≥3 mo[a]	12 mo of negative cultures while on therapy
M kansasii	Rifampin 600 mg by mouth daily or rifabutin 150–300 mg by mouth daily plus Ethambutol 15 mg/kg by mouth daily plus Azithromycin 250 mg by mouth daily or clarithromycin 500 mg by mouth BID or moxifloxacin 400 mg by mouth daily[b]	12 mo of negative cultures while on therapy. In rifampin-resistant M kansasii disease, a 3-drug regimen is recommended based on in vitro susceptibilities
M xenopi	Clarithromycin 500 mg by mouth BID or azithromycin 250 mg by mouth daily plus Isoniazid 300–600 mg by mouth daily plus Rifampin 600 mg by mouth daily or rifabutin 150–300 mg plus Ethambutol 15 mg/kg by mouth daily plus IV streptomycin or amikacin, depending on severity[a]	12 mo of negative cultures while on therapy
M szulgai	Rifampin 600 mg by mouth daily or rifabutin 150–300 mg by mouth daily plus Ethambutol 15 mg/kg by mouth daily plus Azithromycin 250 mg by mouth daily or clarithromycin 500 mg by mouth BID or moxifloxacin 400 mg by mouth daily[b]	12 mo negative cultures on therapy

(continued on next page)

Table 1
(continued)

NTM	Drug Regimen	Duration of Therapy

M malmoense[c]	Rifampin 600 mg by mouth daily
	plus
	Ethambutol 15 mg/kg by mouth daily
	plus
	Isoniazid 300 mg by mouth daily
	plus
	Azithromycin 250 mg by mouth daily or
	  clarithromycin 500 mg by mouth BID
	  or moxifloxacin 400 mg by mouth
	  daily
		2 mo negative cultures on therapy

M simiae[c]	Double-strength Bactrim by mouth BID
	plus
	Amikacin 5–15 mg/kg IV TIW
	plus
	Azithromycin 250 mg by mouth daily or
	  clarithromycin 500 mg by mouth BID
	  or moxifloxacin 400 mg by mouth
	  daily
		12 mo negative cultures on therapy

Abbreviations: BID, twice a day; IM, intramuscularly; IV, intravenously; TIW, 3 times weekly.
[a] Peak levels should be monitored at least weekly.
[b] Isoniazid has traditionally been given in this regimen and is recommended in the 2007 ATS/IDSA guidelines but has questionable value with rifampin and ethambutol and less activity against *M kansasii* compared with newer macrolides and fluoroquinolones.
[c] No therapeutic regimen of proven efficacy.

regimens was an independent predictor of an unfavorable microbiological response. This outcome has not yet been confirmed by others.[33]

Limited data suggest that for patients who do not tolerate rifamycins, clofazimine may provide an effective alternative, combined with ethambutol and a macrolide.[34] Van Ingen and colleagues[35] evaluated 564 clinical NTM isolates, including 16 clinical MAC isolates, for in vitro synergy between amikacin and clofazimine. Significant synergy was reported against all MAC isolates. The investigators concluded that the safety and tolerability of adding clofazimine to amikacin-containing regimens should be tested in clinical trials. The clinical significance of such synergy is not proved. It has been known for many years that the combination of rifampin and ethambutol results in synergistic killing of MAC in vitro, but there is no clear clinical consequence of that observation. Van Ingen and colleagues also noted that the observed in vitro synergy between rifampin and ethambutol is "of questionable clinical significance." The previously cited data from Miwa and colleagues beg the question if a third drug beyond macrolide and ethambutol is even needed for some patients.

Adjunctive surgery for selected patients is associated with favorable treatment outcomes, although surgeons experienced in mycobacterial lung disease remain an important factor for successful outcomes.[36,37] As with drug-resistant tuberculosis, many aspects of surgical management for patients with NTM remain nonstandardized and controversial, including surgical indications, optimal patient selection, and choice of specific surgical procedures.

- Nodular bronchiectasis is typically treated with 3 times weekly dosing of clarithromycin 1000 mg or azithromycin 500 mg, ethambutol 25 mg/kg, and rifampin 600 mg (or rifabutin 150–300 mg), as recommended by the ATS. Dosing adjustments may be required for low body weight and age. Severe cases, including reinfection or relapse, may require the addition of an injectable aminoglycoside. Inhaled amikacin may provide another option for therapy, but care should be taken to ensure that adequate companion drugs are available to prevent the emergence of amikacin resistance.
- A macrolide with a single companion drug, ethambutol, may be adequate for minimal nodular bronchiectatic MAC disease if the patient is intolerant to a rifamycin.
- Patients are considered treatment failures if they have not had a response (microbiological, clinical, or radiographic) after 6 months of appropriate therapy or achieved culture

negativity of sputum after 12 months of therapy.

- Cavitary MAC disease or severe nodular bronchiectatic disease is treated with a daily regimen that includes clarithromycin 500 to 1000 mg/d or azithromycin 250 mg/d, ethambutol 15 mg/kg per day and rifampin 10 mg/kg per day (maximum 600 mg) or rifabutin 150–300 mg/d. Three times weekly therapy may be sufficient, but limited data are available. For patients with cavitary changes on either daily or 3 times weekly oral drugs, amikacin or streptomycin given intravenously or intramuscularly at a dose of approximately 7 to 15 mg/kg 3 times weekly for at least the first 3 months is recommended. Prolonged treatment may be required. The role of inhaled amikacin in this setting is unknown.
- Use of a quinolone and a macrolide without other companion drugs and macrolide monotherapy are not recommended because of poor response and promotion of macrolide resistance. For patients failing standard therapy, the addition of moxifloxacin to multidrug regimens may improve long-term outcome.
- Early specialist referral in patients with severe, refractory, complex, or macrolide-resistant disease is warranted.

Mycobacterium kansasii

M kansasii remains the most easily treatable of the NTM pulmonary pathogens and often presents in a similar manner to reactivation tuberculosis with upper lobe cavitary lesions. As opposed to most other NTM, there is a good correlation between in vitro susceptibility and in vivo response for a variety of antimicrobial agents, including rifamycins, macrolides, and fluoroquinolones. Untreated strains of M kansasii are susceptible to rifamycins (rifampin and rifabutin) with MICs of 1 μg/mL or lesser. Isoniazid and ethambutol are not recommended for reporting by the CLSI, because no broth MIC break points are available. Because of favorable clinical responses associated with in vitro susceptibilities, only rifampin and clarithromycin should be reported, except in rare cases of drug intolerance or in cases in which an M kansasii strain has become rifampin resistant. Should this situation occur, testing of ancillary agents such as amikacin, ethambutol, fluoroquinolones, linezolid, trimethoprim-sulfamethoxazole, tetracyclines, and rifabutin becomes important. The prognosis of even rifampin-resistant M kansasii isolates is good.[14]

A 2003 study by Griffith and colleagues[38] suggested that an intermittent regimen (3 times weekly) of rifampin, ethambutol, and macrolide is effective, less toxic, and less expensive than the standard 18-month daily dosage regimen comprising rifampin, ethambutol, and isoniazid. In the intermittent regimen described, the mean time to sputum conversion to negative culture was less than 2 months. A daily 3-drug regimen comprising rifampin, isoniazid, and ethambutol for a duration including 12 months of sputum culture negativity is recommended for treating M kansasii lung disease. Because of the questionable value of isoniazid in the recommended regimen and because of the excellent activity of the newer macrolides and fluoroquinolones with M kansasii, it is our practice to substitute a newer macrolide or fluoroquinolone for isoniazid. It is also likely that with this strategy, shorter or intermittent treatment regimens for M kansasii lung disease would be successful. It is not clear how a multicenter trial showing the efficacy of a shorter course treatment regimen might be accomplished.

Mycobacterium malmoense

A prospective study of 106 patients with M malmoense lung disease was performed over a 5-year period by the British Thoracic Society (BTS).[39] The results of 2 years of treatment with rifampin plus ethambutol were equivalent to rifampin, ethambutol plus isoniazid, although only 53% of patients were alive at 5 years, and 44 of the original 106 patients (42%) were cured of the infection. In a follow-up study,[40] the BTS randomly assigned 167 patients with M malmoense lung disease to clarithromycin, rifampin, and ethambutol, or ciprofloxacin, rifampin, and ethambutol. Overall response rates were low, but the group receiving clarithromycin had slightly better clinical response and lower mortality. In a retrospective case series from the Netherlands, Hoefsloot and colleagues[41] noted good clinical outcome in 21 of 30 (70%) patients. The success rate was higher in patients receiving isoniazid and rifampin than for patients receiving a macrolide-based regimen. There is no consensus on the optimal treatment regimen for M malmoense, but a regimen including isoniazid, rifampin, and ethambutol with or without a macrolide or fluoroquinolone is tepidly recommended.

Mycobacterium xenopi

M xenopi lung infections have been noted to occur in patients with multiple comorbidities and coinfections and perhaps as a result have high all-cause mortality.[8] One BTS trial[42] reported extremely low 5-year survival rates for patients with M xenopi lung disease (24% treated with rifampin/ethambutol, 10% treated with isoniazid/rifampin/ethambutol); in a second trial,[40] in patients treated with rifampin/ethambutol with either ciprofloxacin or clarithromycin, the regimen including clarithromycin performed slightly better, but mortality and treatment failure rates were still high. In an uncontrolled retrospective study of 136 patients with *M xenopi* pulmonary infection from France,[43] the absence of treatment was associated with a particularly poor prognosis; median survival was 10 months in untreated patients compared with 32 months in treated patients. Combination therapy with a rifamycin-containing regimen was associated with improved survival. These outcomes were not adjusted for comorbidities; therefore, the difference in survival cannot be definitively attributed to treatment. In a similar study from the Netherlands,[44] multiple different treatment regimens were used in 49 patients with *M xenopi* lung disease, but no specific drug combination showed consistently superior results. A recent study of *M xenopi* infection in nude mice[45] found that amikacin-containing regimens were the most effective against *M xenopi*, and no differences were found between regimens containing clarithromycin and oxfloxacin in vivo. An ethambutol/rifampin combination with clarithromycin or moxifloxacin had significant bactericidal activity against *M xenopi*. Although still controversial and lacking conclusive proof of superior efficacy, the ATS/IDSA recommendation for a regimen including rifampin/ethambutol with clarithromycin and adjunctive aminoglycoside initially seems appropriately aggressive, given the high mortality associated with *M xenopi* infection. Although isoniazid is also recommended, it does not seem to add significantly to the other drugs in the regimen.

Mycobacterium szulgai

Although pulmonary *M szulgai* disease is rare, clinical *M szulgai* isolates are generally regarded as clinically significant.[14,46,47] This assertion has recently come into question, which reinforces the need to evaluate all patients with slowly growing NTM disease, according to ATS/IDSA guidelines.[46,47] Disease occurs most commonly in patients with underlying lung disease, such as chronic obstructive lung disease. In 2 studies of patients treated for *M szulgai* infection,[46,47] patients responded well to multiple treatment regimens, usually including rifampin, ethambutol, and either clarithromycin or ciprofloxacin. Patients with *M szulgai* lung disease seem more likely to respond to therapy than patients with *M malmoense*, *M xenopi*, or *M simiae* infection. Given the limited available data, the ATS/IDSA treatment guidelines seem adequate for diagnosis and treatment of *M szulgai* lung disease.[14]

Mycobacterium simiae

M simiae, when isolated in clinical samples, is more often a contaminant than a true pathogen.[14] The clinical presentation, including the typical accompanying symptoms, is usually similar to that of other slow-growing NTM associated with nodular bronchiectatic disease. *M simiae* can also be associated with a more rapidly progressive cavitary form of disease.

As a true pathogen, *M simiae* is difficult to treat effectively. Among the many difficult to treat slowly growing NTM pathogens, *M simiae* holds the dubious honor of being the most difficult. There are no predictably effective drug combinations for treating *M simiae*.[48–50] A multidrug regimen based on susceptibility testing is recommended for this multidrug-resistant organism; however, many *M simiae* isolates show in vitro susceptibility to amikacin only or perhaps amikacin plus sulfa, leaving the clinician in a quandary about how to cobble together an effective regimen. Some experts recommend parenteral amikacin-based regimens, with some combination of sulfa, fluoroquinolone, macrolide, and linezolid, regardless of the in vitro susceptibilities. *M simiae* clearly presents a great challenge, with little guidance for treatment other than anecdotal experience.

NONPHARMACOLOGIC TREATMENT OPTIONS

Mounting evidence suggests that household sources of NTM exposure, specifically household plumbing and water sources, are important for contracting NTM pathogens. The recent evidence of likely NTM recurrence after successful NTM therapy in bronchiectasis suggests an ongoing host vulnerability, which seems to suggest the necessity for efforts to limit environmental NTM exposure.[25] However, it is still unknown how much of a risk NTM in municipal water and household plumbing presents for most patients with bronchiectasis and NTM lung disease. It is also not certain, for instance, that avoidance of aerosolized water from showers without avoidance of other potential aerosol-generating activities associated with running water in the home would eliminate the risk of household NTM transmission. Interventions such as increasing the temperature of the hot water heater to $\geq 54.4°C$ ($\geq 130°F$) or changing shower heads at regular intervals might decrease risk of NTM transmission, but the impact of these steps is not known.[51] Moreover, limited experience suggests that cleaning shower heads with bleach may not result in sustained decreased exposure risk to NTM over time, so that no clear recommendations can be made regarding the efficacy or optimal timing of regular cleaning of shower heads with bleach. It is also still unknown whether exposure to specific soil-based sources of NTM organisms may contribute to the development of NTM lung disease.[52]

Because NTM exposure is ubiquitous and NTM lung disease is uncommon, the development of NTM lung disease in most circumstances must require a combination of environmental exposure and host susceptibility. Bronchiectasis and pulmonary NTM infection are unquestionably and inextricably linked. Patients with CF are at high risk of pulmonary NTM infection, which strongly supports the role of a predisposing alteration in airway-surface defenses for the acquisition of NTM infection. Prevots and colleagues[6] reported a nested case control study of 48 patients with CF with NTM lung disease and 85 controls without NTM infection to evaluate possible associations between NTM lung disease and environmental exposure. These investigators found that indoor swimming was associated with incident NTM infection, although only a few patients in each group had indoor swimming pools. Average annual atmospheric water vapor content was also significantly predictive of prevalence of NTM lung infection in CF centers. Exposure to showering and municipal water supply was not different between the infected and uninfected groups. The investigators believed that because exposure to NTM is ubiquitous and behaviors are similar among persons with and without pulmonary NTM disease, genetic susceptibility beyond CF is likely important for NTM disease development.

There is no evidence to support any role for dietary changes, such as avoidance of cheese, in the treatment of MAC lung disease. Maintaining adequate caloric intake, body mass index, and following prealbumin levels as a marker of nutrition may be helpful. Some individuals also find it helpful to take probiotic therapy while taking an antibiotic regimen for NTM disease.

Exercise, including pulmonary rehabilitation, is encouraged in individuals with chronic lung disease, but this has not been studied in NTM lung disease. Aerobic activity and deep breathing activities such as yoga are generally believed to be helpful.

Cessation of cigarette smoking is essential.

TREATMENT RESISTANCE/COMPLICATIONS

An additional critical element in the management of patients with MAC lung disease is prevention of the emergence of macrolide resistance. Although the role of in vitro susceptibility for most other agents remains controversial, it is clear that the development of macrolide resistance in a MAC isolate (MIC >16 μg/mL) is strongly associated with treatment failure and increased mortality.[31] The most important risk factors for developing macrolide-resistant MAC are macrolide monotherapy and the combination of macrolide and fluoroquinolone without a third companion drug.

Recent data have been published regarding the benefits of the use of macrolide monotherapy to decrease rates of exacerbations in patients with chronic obstructive pulmonary disease (COPD) and non–CF-related bronchiectasis.[53,54] Increasing interest and ongoing multicenter studies are hoping to answer whether there may be a role for macrolide monotherapy to improve the natural course of adult patients who have non-CF bronchiectasis. The relative tolerance and potential benefit raise complex questions grounded in the relationship between bronchiectasis and NTM lung disease, as well as the deleterious risk of creating macrolide-resistant NTM lung disease, as discussed earlier. Without clear data or recommendations available to direct the clinician, a common approach to the adult patient with non-CF bronchiectasis is similar to the patient with CF and macrolide monotherapy. Specifically, before consideration of the start of macrolide monotherapy, NTM lung disease should be excluded on clinical, radiographic, and as appropriate, microbiological criteria. Caution should be exercised before starting macrolide monotherapy in those adult patients with non-CF bronchiectasis with past history of NTM lung disease, given the real possibility of subsequent relapse or reinfection with the same or different NTM organism and risk of creating macrolide-resistant NTM lung disease. The use of macrolide monotherapy in those with established macrolide-resistant NTM lung disease for immunomodulatory purposes is also undefined but at least superficially seems to be justifiable.

MAC in vitro resistance to amikacin is associated with a specific 16S ribosomal RNA mutation and an MIC to amikacin greater than 64 μg/mL. Perhaps more significant, the mutation conferring resistance and the high MIC were associated with poor clinical response and treatment failure. These observations suggest that amikacin is the second drug other than macrolide in which in vitro susceptibility correlates with in vivo response in the treatment of MAC lung disease.[55] If this finding is correct, it places a burden on clinicians to make sure that amikacin is administered with adequate companion medications to prevent the emergence of mutational resistance to amikacin. It also raises the question of whether inhaled amikacin would be more likely to induce mutational resistance then parenteral amikacin.

EVALUATION OF OUTCOME AND LONG-TERM RECOMMENDATIONS

Long-term follow-up is essential in NTM lung disease. We recommend monthly sputum sampling for AFB as well as routine culture while patients are taking antibiotic therapy and every 1 to 2 months thereafter after cessation of therapy, at the least for the first year after stopping antimicrobials. Although there are no established guidelines, we obtain imaging by chest radiograph and high-resolution computed tomography (CT) of the chest before starting therapy for NTM. Repeat radiographs, usually chest radiographs, are obtained at a minimum approximately every 2 months after initiating therapy and at the cessation of antibiotic therapy. Most subspecialists agree that when considering repeat CT scans, the long-term consequences of relatively high radiation exposure and accumulated radiation dose should be considered by the medical team. As with all tests, a risk/benefit balance should be considered for each test. Our approach is to limit CT scans on a routine basis to initiation and completion of therapy, with scans requested during therapy if there is a specific question that can only be answered with a CT scan. Patients are more aware of radiation exposure and frequently question the need for CT scans. Clinical symptoms must be followed to identify response to therapy and the potential for relapse or reinfection in the treated patient.

SUMMARY

Slowly growing mycobacteria cause most NTM lung disease in the United States, with MAC the most frequent and important NTM pulmonary pathogen. Treatment of MAC is usually successful, although not as often successful as treatment of tuberculosis. Guideline-based therapy is effective, although for unclear reasons, it is not embraced for many patients with MAC lung disease. The consequence of inadequate MAC therapy can be the emergence of macrolide-resistant MAC, which is associated with high rates of treatment failure and increased mortality. Treatment of M kansasii lung disease is simple and usually successful. Treatment regimens for other slowly growing NTM are not well established and require clinical judgment on the part of the treating physician. M xenopi disease deserves special attention because of high mortality with this pathogen. M simiae is difficult to treat successfully and lacks any predictably effective treatment regimen. Overall, successful antibiotic therapy for slowly growing NTM pathogens should be guided by an experienced physician and should comprise an adequate number of drugs based on appropriate susceptibility testing.

REFERENCES

1. Griffith DE, Aksamit TR. Bronchiectasis and nontuberculous mycobacterial disease. Clin Chest Med 2012;33:283–95.
2. Kim RD, Greenberg DE, Ehrmantraut ME, et al. Pulmonary nontuberculous mycobacterial disease: prospective study of a distinct preexisting syndrome. Am J Respir Crit Care Med 2008;178:1066–74.
3. Kartalija M, Ovrutsky AR, Bryan CL, et al. Patients with nontuberculous mycobacterial lung disease exhibit unique body and immune phenotypes. Am J Respir Crit Care Med 2013;187:197–205.
4. Mai HN, Hijikata M, Inoue Y, et al. Pulmonary *Mycobacterium avium* complex infection associated with the IVS8-T5 allele of the CFTR gene. Int J Tuberc Lung Dis 2007;11:808–13.
5. Bienvenu T, Sermet-Gaudelus I, Burgel PR, et al. Cystic fibrosis transmembrane conductance regulator channel dysfunction in non-cystic fibrosis bronchiectasis. Am J Respir Crit Care Med 2010;181:1078–84.
6. Prevots DR, Adjemian J, Fernandez AG, et al. Environmental risks for nontuberculous mycobacteria: individual exposures and climatic factors in the cystic fibrosis population. Ann Am Thorac Soc 2014;11(7):1032–8.
7. Adjemian J, Olivier KN, Prevots DR. Nontuberculous mycobacteria among cystic fibrosis patients in the United States: screening practices and environmental risk. Am J Respir Crit Care Med 2014; 190(5):581–6.
8. van Ingen J, Ferro BE, Hoefsloot W, et al. Drug treatment of pulmonary nontuberculous mycobacterial disease in HIV-negative patients: the evidence. Expert Rev Anti Infect Ther 2013;11:1065–77.
9. Carrillo MC, Patsios D, Wagnetz U, et al. Comparison of the spectrum of radiologic and clinical manifestations of pulmonary disease caused by *Mycobacterium avium* complex and *Mycobacterium xenopi*. Can Assoc Radiol J 2014;65:207–13.
10. Hayashi M, Takayanagi N, Kanauchi T, et al. Prognostic factors of 634 HIV-negative patients with *Mycobacterium avium* complex lung disease. Am J Respir Crit Care Med 2012;185:575–83.
11. Ito Y, Hirai T, Maekawa K, et al. Predictors of 5-year mortality in pulmonary *Mycobacterium avium-intracellulare* complex disease. Int J Tuberc Lung Dis 2012;16(3):408–14.
12. Shu CC, Lee CH, Hsu CL, et al. Clinical characteristics and prognosis of nontuberculous mycobacterial

lung disease with different radiographic patterns. Lung 2011;189:467–74.

13. Kitada S, Uenami T, Yoshimura K, et al. Long-term radiographic outcome of nodular bronchiectatic *Mycobacterium avium* complex pulmonary disease. Int J Tuberc Lung Dis 2012;16:660–4.

14. Griffith DE, Aksamit T, Brown-Elliott BA, et al. An official ATS/IDSA statement: diagnosis, treatment, and prevention of nontuberculous mycobacterial diseases. Am J Respir Crit Care Med 2007;175: 367–416.

15. Woods G, Brown-Elliott B, Conville PS, et al. Susceptibility testing of mycobacteria, nocardiae, and other aerobic actinomycetes; approved standard. 2nd edition. Wayne, PA: Clinical and Laboratory Standards Institute (CLSI); 2003. CLSI document M24–A2.

16. Kobashi Y, Yoshida K, Miyashita N, et al. Relationship between clinical efficacy of treatment of pulmonary *Mycobacterium avium* complex disease and drug-sensitivity testing of *Mycobacterium avium* complex isolates. J Infect Chemother 2006;12:195–202.

17. Wallace RJ Jr, Brown BA, Griffith DE, et al. Clarithromycin regimens for pulmonary *Mycobacterium avium* complex. The first 50 patients. Am J Respir Crit Care Med 1996;153:1766–72.

18. Griffith DE, Brown BA, Girard WM, et al. Azithromycin activity against *Mycobacterium avium* complex lung disease in patients who were not infected with human immunodeficiency virus. Clin Infect Dis 1996;23:983–9.

19. Tanaka E, Kimoto T, Tsuyuguchi K, et al. Effect of clarithromycin regimen for *Mycobacterium avium* complex pulmonary disease. Am J Respir Crit Care Med 1999;160:866–72.

20. van Ingen J, Boeree MJ, van Soolingen D, et al. Resistance mechanisms and drug susceptibility testing of nontuberculous mycobacteria. Drug Resist Updat 2012;15:149–61.

21. van Ingen J, Egelund EF, Levin A, et al. The pharmacokinetics and pharmacodynamics of pulmonary *Mycobacterium avium* complex disease treatment. Am J Respir Crit Care Med 2012;186:559–65.

22. Dheda K, Shean K, Zumla A, et al. Early treatment outcomes and HIV status of patients with extensively drug-resistant tuberculosis in South Africa: a retrospective cohort study. Lancet 2010;375: 1798–807.

23. Adjemian J, Prevots DR, Gallagher J, et al. Lack of adherence to evidence-based treatment guidelines for nontuberculous mycobacterial lung disease. Ann Am Thorac Soc 2014;11:9–16.

24. Marras TK, Prevots DR, Jamieson FB, et al, Pulmonary MAC Outcomes Group. Opinions differ by expertise in *Mycobacterium avium* complex disease. Ann Am Thorac Soc 2014;11:17–22.

25. Wallace RJ Jr, Brown-Elliott BA, McNulty S, et al. Macrolide/azalide therapy for nodular/bronchiectatic: *Mycobacterium avium* complex lung disease. Chest 2014;146(2):276–82.

26. Miwa S, Shirai M, Toyoshima M, et al. Efficacy of clarithromycin and ethambutol for *Mycobacterium avium* complex pulmonary disease. A preliminary study. Ann Am Thorac Soc 2014;11:23–9.

27. Davis KK, Kao PN, Jacobs SS, et al. Aerosolized amikacin for treatment of pulmonary *Mycobacterium avium* infections: an observational case series. BMC Pulm Med 2007;7:2.

28. Olivier KN, Shaw PA, Glaser TS, et al. Inhaled amikacin for treatment of refractory pulmonary nontuberculous mycobacterial disease. Ann Am Thorac Soc 2014;11:30–5.

29. Olivier KN, Gupta R, Daley CL et al. A controlled study of liposomal amikacin for inhalation in patients with recalcitrant nontuberculous mycobacterial lung disease. Abstract #50985, Presented at the annual meeting of the American Thoracic Society. San Diego, May 16–21, 2014.

30. Rao GA, Mann JR, Shoaibi A, et al. Azithromycin and levofloxacin use and increased risk of cardiac arrhythmia and death. Ann Fam Med 2014; 12:121–7.

31. Griffith DE, Brown-Elliott BA, Langsjoen B, et al. Clinical and molecular analysis of macrolide resistance in *Mycobacterium avium* complex lung disease. Am J Respir Crit Care Med 2006;174:928–34.

32. Koh WJ, Hong G, Kim SY, et al. Treatment of refractory *Mycobacterium avium* complex lung disease with a moxifloxacin-containing regimen. Antimicrob Agents Chemother 2013;57:2281–5.

33. Jo KW, Kim S, Lee JY, et al. Treatment outcomes of refractory MAC pulmonary disease treated with drugs with unclear efficacy. J Infect Chemother 2014;20(10):602–6.

34. Field SK, Cowie RL. Treatment of *Mycobacterium avium-intracellulare* complex lung disease with a macrolide, ethambutol, and clofazimine. Chest 2003;124:1482–6.

35. van Ingen J, Totten SE, Helstrom NK, et al. In vitro synergy between clofazimine and amikacin in treatment of nontuberculous mycobacterial disease. Antimicrob Agents Chemother 2012;56: 6324–7.

36. Mitchell JD, Yu JA, Bishop A, et al. Thoracoscopic lobectomy and segmentectomy for infectious lung disease. Ann Thorac Surg 2012;93:1033–9 [discussion: 1039–40].

37. Yu JA, Pomerantz M, Bishop A, et al. Lady Windermere revisited: treatment with thoracoscopic lobectomy/segmentectomy for right middle lobe and lingular bronchiectasis associated with nontuberculous mycobacterial disease. Eur J Cardiothorac Surg 2011;40:671–5.

38. Griffith DE, Brown-Elliott BA, Wallace RJ Jr. Thrice-weekly clarithromycin-containing regimen for treatment of *Mycobacterium kansasii* lung disease: results of a preliminary study. Clin Infect Dis 2003; 37:1178–82.

39. Pulmonary disease caused by *M. malmoense* in HIV negative patients: 5-yr follow-up of patients receiving standardised treatment. Eur Respir J 2003; 21:478–82.

40. Jenkins PA, Campbell IA, Banks J, et al. Clarithromycin vs ciprofloxacin as adjuncts to rifampicin and ethambutol in treating opportunist mycobacterial lung diseases and an assessment of *Mycobacterium vaccae* immunotherapy. Thorax 2008;63:627–34.

41. Hoefsloot W, van Ingen J, de Lange WC, et al. Clinical relevance of *Mycobacterium malmoense* isolation in The Netherlands. Eur Respir J 2009; 34:926–31.

42. Research Committee of the British Thoracic Society. First randomised trial of treatments for pulmonary disease caused by *M avium intracellulare*, *M malmoense*, and *M xenopi* in HIV negative patients: rifampicin, ethambutol and isoniazid versus rifampicin and ethambutol. Thorax 2001;56:167–72.

43. Andrejak C, Lescure FX, Pukenyte E, et al. *Mycobacterium xenopi* pulmonary infections: a multicentric retrospective study of 136 cases in north-east France. Thorax 2009;64:291–6.

44. van Ingen J, Boeree MJ, de Lange WC, et al. *Mycobacterium xenopi* clinical relevance and determinants, the Netherlands. Emerg Infect Dis 2008;14: 385–9.

45. Andrejak C, Almeida DV, Tyagi S, et al. Improving existing tools for *Mycobacterium xenopi* treatment: assessment of drug combinations and characterization of mouse models of infection and chemotherapy. J Antimicrob Chemother 2013;68: 659–65.

46. Yoo H, Jeon K, Kim SY, et al. Clinical significance of *Mycobacterium szulgai* isolates from respiratory specimens. Scand J Infect Dis 2014;46:169–74.

47. van Ingen J, Boeree MJ, de Lange WC, et al. Clinical relevance of *Mycobacterium szulgai* in The Netherlands. Clin Infect Dis 2008;46:1200–5.

48. van Ingen J, Boeree MJ, Dekhuijzen PN, et al. Clinical relevance of *Mycobacterium simiae* in pulmonary samples. Eur Respir J 2008;31:106–9.

49. Valero G, Moreno F, Graybill JR. Activities of clarithromycin, ofloxacin, and clarithromycin plus ethambutol against *Mycobacterium simiae* in murine model of disseminated infection. Antimicrob Agents Chemother 1994;38:2676–7.

50. Valero G, Peters J, Jorgensen JH, et al. Clinical isolates of *Mycobacterium simiae* in San Antonio, Texas. An 11-yr review. Am J Respir Crit Care Med 1995;152:1555–7.

51. Falkinham JO 3rd. Nontuberculous mycobacteria from household plumbing of patients with nontuberculous mycobacteria disease. Emerg Infect Dis 2011;17:419–24.

52. Fujita K, Ito Y, Hirai T, et al. Association between polyclonal and mixed mycobacterial *Mycobacterium avium* complex infection and environmental exposure. Ann Am Thorac Soc 2014;11:45–53.

53. Albert RK, Connett J, Bailey WC, et al. Azithromycin for prevention of exacerbations of COPD. N Engl J Med 2011;365:689–98.

54. Wong C, Jayaram L, Karalus N, et al. Azithromycin for prevention of exacerbations in non-cystic fibrosis bronchiectasis (EMBRACE): a randomised, double-blind, placebo-controlled trial. Lancet 2012;380:660–7.

55. Brown-Elliott BA, Iakhiaeva E, Griffith DE, et al. In vitro activity of amikacin against isolates of *Mycobacterium avium* complex with proposed MIC breakpoints and finding of a 16S rRNA gene mutation in treated isolates. J Clin Microbiol 2013;51:3389–94.

Nontuberculous Mycobacteria Infections in Immunosuppressed Hosts

Emily Henkle, PhD, MPH[a],*, Kevin L. Winthrop, MD, MPH[b,c]

KEYWORDS

- *Mycobacterium avium* • Extrapulmonary nontuberculous mycobacteria • Transplant
- Immunosuppressive therapy

KEY POINTS

- Nontuberculous mycobacteria (NTM) disease is an important cause of disease in immunosuppressed hosts.
- *Mycobacterium avium* complex is the leading cause of NTM disease in immunosuppressed patients, but rapid growers including *Mycobacterium abscessus*, *Mycobacterium chelonae*, *Mycobacterium fortuitum*, and a variety of rare species are also important.
- In immunosuppressed patients, about half of NTM disease is pulmonary and the remainder is split between skin/soft tissue and disseminated.
- Treatment is species specific and requires expert management with the ability to cure such infections related to the host's underlying immunosuppressive status.

INTRODUCTION

Nontuberculous mycobacteria (NTM) are important causes of pulmonary and extrapulmonary disease in immunosuppressed hosts. Early descriptions of NTM in immunosuppressed hosts come from the cancer literature: in 1976 an institutional report described 30 NTM infections, comprising half of 59 mycobacterial infections in patients with cancer over a 5-year period.[1] Then, in the 1980s, disseminated *Mycobacterium avium* complex (MAC) disease was identified as an important pathogen in the setting of AIDS, highlighting the risk of these environmental organisms within the severely immunocompromised host.[2,3] Simultaneously NTM cases were reported in reviews of mycobacterial disease in renal transplant patients, although tuberculosis was the focus, with poorer patient outcomes.[4,5] Other case reports focusing on NTM disease appeared in the cancer literature.[6–8] Since that time, tuberculosis has declined significantly in the United States; formal population-based epidemiologic studies have demonstrated the burden and increasing incidence of NTM infections, and further described the clinical and epidemiologic risk factors for these infections.[9–13] Although MAC continues to cause most NTM disease in the setting of immunosuppression, it is likely that changes within laboratory diagnostics, the host, and the environment have contributed to an increasingly diverse array of NTM species now being recognized as being associated with immunosuppressive states. This array includes rapidly growing NTM (*Mycobacterium abscessus*, *Mycobacterium chelonae*,

Disclosures: None.

[a] HIV, STD, and TB Section, Public Health Division, Oregon Health Authority, 800 NE Oregon Street, Suite 1105, Portland, OR 97232, USA; [b] Division of Infectious Diseases, Oregon Health and Science University, 3375 Southwest Terwilliger Boulevard, Mailstop CEI, Portland, OR 97239, USA; [c] Division of Public Health and Preventative Medicine, Oregon Health and Science University, 3375 Southwest Terwilliger Boulevard, Mailstop CEI, Portland, OR 97239, USA
* Corresponding author.
E-mail address: emhenkle@gmail.com

Clin Chest Med 36 (2015) 91–99
http://dx.doi.org/10.1016/j.ccm.2014.11.002
0272-5231/15/$ – see front matter © 2015 Elsevier Inc. All rights reserved.

Mycobacterium fortuitum), in addition to species that are difficult to grow in culture whereby molecular techniques might increase their identification (eg, *Mycobacterium haemophilum*). Furthermore, changes in the prevalence of immunosuppression have also likely contributed to these changing trends in NTM disease. The introduction of highly active antiretroviral therapy (HAART) diminished the importance of MAC in the setting of human immunodeficiency virus (HIV), while increasing use of organ transplantation, particularly stem cell transplants, and the widespread use of new biologics and other immunosuppressive therapies for patients with immune-mediated inflammatory disease, has increased the number of patients susceptible to NTM infection. This review discusses the changing landscape of NTM in the immunosuppressed setting, and highlights the particular challenges of NTM prevention and management for immunosuppressed patients.

DISEASE DESCRIPTION

NTM disease is increasing in the United States. Prevots and colleagues[11] used data from several large health maintenance organizations in the western United States and found an increase of 2.6% per year from 1994 to 2006. The first incidence estimate of NTM disease is 5.7 per 100,000 in Oregon in 2012, with rates 3 to 4 times higher in individuals older than 70 years.[14] Most of this is pulmonary disease whereby a large proportion occurs outside of recognized settings of immunosuppression. For others, however, immunosuppression contributes to the risk of acquisition or progression and death. This situation has been described in institutional-based cohorts of patients with cancer or undergoing solid organ or stem cell transplants. More recent population-based studies have confirmed that NTM disease is associated with oral and inhaled corticosteroids associated with chronic obstructive pulmonary disease or biological therapies for immune-mediated inflammatory diseases.[13,15] A recent study of comorbid factors associated with 2990 NTM-related deaths from 1999 to 2010 using death certificate data found that 2% were associated with primary immune deficiency, 1.1% with lymphoma and hematologic malignancies, and 0.5% with HIV.[16]

In general, the underlying mechanism that increases the risk of NTM disease in immunosuppressed patients is disruption or depletion of cell-mediated immunity, a critical component of host defense against mycobacteria. Mycobacteria infect macrophages and stimulate the $CD4^+$ T-helper 1 (TH1) pathway, which involves interleukin (IL)-12 and interferon (IFN)-γ. IFN-γ then activates infected macrophages, which control infection. Another key mechanism of control is via tumor necrosis factor (TNF)-α, a proinflammatory cytokine required for formation and maintenance of granulomas that effectively inhibit bacterial growth.[17] Most of the research into the mechanisms of infection and immunologic control has been conducted on *Mycobacterium tuberculosis*, *Mycobacterium bovis*, and *M avium*. However, it is clear that there are differences in virulence and immune response to different species, evidenced by species variations in the predominant site of infection and the fact that several species, including *M haemophilum* and *Mycobacterium genavense*, cause infection almost exclusively in immunocompromised patients.[18–20] The various settings of immunosuppression that are related to NTM infection are summarized in **Table 1** and are described in more detail in their respective sections.

In immunocompetent patients, approximately 77% of NTM disease is pulmonary.[9] In immunosuppressed patients this proportion ranges from less than 5% in AIDS patients to 67% in patients on biological therapies for immune-mediated inflammatory diseases, with a corresponding increase in disseminated and skin (including surgical-site or catheter-related) infection (see **Table 1**).[21,22] MAC is the most common species for pulmonary and disseminated NTM infection, followed by *M abscessus*, *Mycobacterium kansasii* (found in the Southern and Midwestern United States and internationally), and *Mycobacterium xenopi* (Northern United States and Canada).[23] Rapidly growing NTM, including *M fortuitum*, *M abscessus*, *M chelonae*, *Mycobacterium mucogenicum*, and *Mycobacterium neoaurum*, are causes of skin and catheter-related infection and bacteremia.[24,25] NTM species and typical sites of infection are listed in **Table 2**.

NONTUBERCULOUS MYCOBACTERIA INFECTION BY UNDERLYING DISEASE OR TREATMENT
Human Immunodeficiency Virus/AIDS

Epidemiology
The epidemic of disseminated MAC infection began in 1982 with a sharp increase in the number of cases associated with the AIDS epidemic.[3] Up to 24% of AIDS patients had disseminated MAC by 1989/1990.[2] Distinguishing it from other opportunistic infections that occurred earlier in the course of HIV infection, disseminated MAC was associated with very low $CD4^+$ counts, generally fewer than 50 cells/mm^3.[2,3] The introduction of

Table 1
Immunosuppressive conditions and risks for nontuberculous mycobacteria (NTM)

Underlying Disease or Treatment	No. of NTM Cases in Included References	Pulmonary (%)	Disseminated (%)	Skin/Soft Tissue/ Catheter (%)	Overall Risk/ Relative Risk (RR)	References
AIDS	972		(100)		24%	2
Hairy cell leukemia	9		(100)		5%	56
Hematopoietic stem cell transplant	97	18	9	70	0.4–4.9	48,53,62
Hematologic malignancies	34	76	24		1.2%	55
Solid organ transplant	40	50	15	35	0.02 (various organs) 1.1 (lung) per 100 person-years	49,51
Biological therapy for immune-mediated inflammatory diseases	123	56–67	8	35	74/100,000	15,25
Corticosteroid therapy for chronic respiratory disease	182	(100)			RR Oral: 8 Inhaled: 24.3	13,34

HAART in 1997 led to a sharp decline in the number of disseminated MAC cases.[26,27] *M kansasii* also causes disseminated NTM infection, but causes pulmonary disease in more than half of AIDS patients.[21,23] Post-HAART population data on disseminated NTM has been reported in Oregon, with a published rate of 0.3 per 100,000 in 2005-2006 remaining stable at 0.2 per 100,000 in 2012 (unpublished data by Henkle E, 2014).[9] This figure suggests that the rate of disseminated NTM in the setting of HIV is low, at least in Oregon.

It is unknown as to what proportion of the 9 cases in 2012 had coexistent HIV/AIDS. However, if all of these were assumed to be AIDS related, using the statewide 2012 estimate of 5500 people living in Oregon with HIV as a denominator the proportion of HIV/AIDS patients with disseminated NTM in Oregon was less than 0.2% in 2012.[28]

HIV-related pulmonary disease is still poorly understood. Even in countries where tuberculosis is endemic, NTM may cause significant disease in HIV-infected patients. In Thailand and Vietnam,

Table 2
Nontuberculous *Mycobacterium* species and common sites of infection in immunosuppressed hosts

	Pulmonary	Disseminated	Skin/Soft Tissue/Catheter
Slow growers	MAC *M kansasii* *M xenopi* *M malmoense*	MAC *M kansasii* *M haemophilum* *M marinum* *M genavense* (R)	MAC *M marinum* *M haemophilum* (R)
Rapid growers	*M abscessus*	*M chelonae* *M abscessus* (R) *M fortuitum* (R)	*M abscessus* *M chelonae* *M fortuitum* *M mucogenicum* (R)

Abbreviations: MAC, *M avium/intracellulare* complex; (R), rare.
Adapted from Griffith DE, Aksamit T, Brown-Elliott BA, et al. An official ATS/IDSA statement: diagnosis, treatment, and prevention of nontuberculous mycobacterial diseases. Am J Respir Crit Care Med 2007;175(4):367–416.

NTM disease prevalence was 2% among HIV-infected patients enrolled and screened for mycobacterial infections.[29] Half of these infections were classified as pulmonary and half as disseminated. The cases with pulmonary disease and negative blood cultures generally had typical NTM imaging, including nodules, cavity disease, or infiltrate, suggesting that disease might be related to other underlying lung diseases, similar to what is seen in the non-HIV setting.

Diagnosis, prevention, and treatment

Initially rifabutin prophylaxis was recommended if CD4[+] counts dropped below 50 cells/mm[3], but this was changed to azithromycin or clarithromycin after clinical trials showed their effectiveness.[30] In 2002, after the introduction of HAART, the recommendation was made to discontinue prophylactic antibiotics if HIV disease was well controlled.[27] At present, prophylactic treatment with azithromycin 1200 mg once weekly is recommended for HIV-infected patients with CD4[+] counts lower than 50 cells/mm[3].[23]

Treatment of disseminated MAC includes antivirals to control the underlying immunosuppression in addition to therapy for the NTM infection. The optimal regimen against disseminated MAC is clarithromycin, ethambutol, ± rifabutin (**Table 3**),

based on randomized clinical trials.[23] Rifabutin is often added as the third antibiotic, although the additional benefit of this drug is less established. Untreated disseminated MAC was shown to shorten the time to death in AIDS patients, but treated patients had similar survival compared with non-MAC matched controls.[31] A study of HIV-infected patients hospitalized at a single hospital showed a 10% mortality rate among 19 patients hospitalized for disseminated NTM infection.[32]

IMMUNOSUPPRESSIVE THERAPIES FOR IMMUNE-MEDIATED INFLAMMATORY DISEASES

Corticosteroids

Oral and inhaled corticosteroids are routinely prescribed to suppress inflammation in several chronic conditions, including chronic obstructive pulmonary disease (COPD), asthma, and rheumatoid arthritis. Corticosteroids are known to increase the risk of pneumonia in patients with COPD and tuberculosis as much as 5-fold,[33] while the relative risks of NTM are likely even greater. Oral prednisone use was 8 times higher among NTM cases than in controls in a case-control study in Oregon and Washington.[34] Inhaled

Table 3
Preferred treatment regimens for nontuberculous mycobacteria as per 2007 ATS/IDSA guidelines

Disease Site/Species	Drug Combination[a,b]	Susceptibility Testing
Pulmonary M avium (nodular)	Macrolide + ethambutol + rifampin	Recommended for macrolides
Pulmonary M avium (cavitary, severe, previously treated)	Above + IV/IM streptomycin or amikacin	Recommended for macrolides
Disseminated M avium complex	Clarithromycin + ethambutol + rifabutin	Recommended for macrolides
Pulmonary M kansasii	Rifampin + ethambutol + isoniazid + pyridoxine	Recommended for rifampin
M abscessus	Macrolide[c] + 1 or more of IV amikacin, cefoxitin, or imipenem	Recommended for a panel of drugs
M chelonae	Multidrug therapies including clarithromycin	Recommended for a panel of drugs
M fortuitum	Multidrug therapies including clarithromycin[c]	Recommended for a panel of drugs
M haemophilum	Multidrug from clarithromycin, rifabutin/rifampin, ciprofloxacin	Recommended (interpret with caution)

Abbreviations: ATS, American Thoracic Society; IDSA, Infectious Disease Society of America; IM, intramuscular; IV, intravenous.
[a] Oral unless noted.
[b] Treatment length minimum 12 months culture negative (pulmonary), 4 to 6 months (skin/soft tissue).
[c] M abscessus subspecies abscessus and M fortuitum have an erm gene that can result in inducible macrolide resistance in the presence of a macrolide. Therefore, these drugs may not be affective in the treatment of infections caused by these organisms.
Data from Griffith DE, Aksamit T, Brown-Elliott BA, et al. An official ATS/IDSA statement: diagnosis, treatment, and prevention of nontuberculous mycobacterial diseases. Am J Respir Crit Care Med 2007;175:367–416.

corticosteroids were associated with a significantly increased NTM risk of 24.3 in a study of COPD patients in Denmark.[13] Asthmatic NTM cases had a longer duration and higher dose of inhaled corticosteroids compared with controls in a Japanese case-control study.[35] In all 3 studies there was a clear dose response, with higher risks of NTM with oral prednisone doses greater than 15 mg and greater than 800 mg fluticasone equivalent.

Biological Therapy

TNF-α is a proinflammatory cytokine that is integral to host defense against granulomatous mycobacterial and fungal infections.[36–38] Medications that target the TNF pathway are the cornerstone of the treatment of autoimmune inflammatory conditions including rheumatoid arthritis, psoriasis, and Crohn disease. Five TNF-α inhibitors are currently approved: infliximab, adalimumab, golimumab, and certolizumab are anti–TNF-α monoclonal antibodies, and etanercept is a soluble receptor fusion protein.[39] In a United States study of new users of infliximab, etanercept, or adalimumab anti-TNF therapy, the overall rates of NTM disease were 5- to 10-fold higher than disease rates seen in the unexposed background rheumatoid arthritis and general populations, and more common than tuberculosis.[15] The drug-specific incidence rates per 100,000 patient-years and 95% confidence intervals were 35 (1–69) for etanercept, 116 (30–203) for infliximab, and 122 (3–241) for adalimumab. In South Korea a higher incidence of NTM disease of 230 per 100,000 patients was reported in 2 separate hospital-based reviews of 509 and 1165 patients treated with TNF antagonists.[40,41] In a review of US Food and Drug Administration MedWatch reports, just over half (55%) of NTM cases were pulmonary.[25] In the United States and South Korea, 70% to 100% of NTM infections were in patients with rheumatoid arthritis, who frequently have associated underlying lung disease including bronchiectasis and interstitial lung disease.[15,25,41,42]

Other biological agents used in this setting include rituximab (anti-CD20 monoclonal antibody), abatacept (T-cell costimulator modulator), tocilizumab (anti–IL-6 monoclonal antibody), and ustekinumab (anti–IL-12 monoclonal antibody). There is a theoretic increased risk of NTM infection with these agents, but few safety data exist and further study is required.[39] At present, the evidence of NTM risk is limited to small case series of NTM disease in patients treated with rituximab (2 cases) and tocilizumab (4 cases; 3 were also taking prednisolone ± tacrolimus and 2 had prior NTM infection).[43,44] It should be noted that rituximab has been used as an adjunct to successfully treat otherwise recalcitrant chronic NTM infections in patients with autoantibody states involving IFN-γ.[45,46]

Diagnosis, Prevention, and Treatment

Prospective screening is not recommended for any of the immunosuppressed groups, unlike tuberculosis whereby there are clear benefits to screening for latent infection before the initiation of biologics and immunosuppressive therapy.[23] However, some groups should be considered for further clinical workup before initiation of biological therapy. Patients with chronic cough that cannot be explained by usual causes should be considered for further workup for pulmonary NTM, including computed tomography imaging and respiratory sampling.

Treatment is described in **Table 3** and is species specific, requiring antimicrobial susceptibility for all except MAC, unless macrolide-resistant MAC is suspected.[23] When possible, decreasing or dropping immunosuppressive medications likely improves the likelihood of successful treatment.[38] Nonbiologics such as methotrexate should be considered, or second-line therapies such as abatacept or tocilizumab, which are currently considered lower risk.[15] Outcomes of pulmonary disease treatment are variable. Case fatality rates range from less than 10% to 15% in United States studies with short-term follow-up. Winthrop and colleagues[15] reported a higher case fatality rate of 39% with a median of 569 days (range 21–2127) between diagnosis and death. Evidence from a small Japanese case series suggests that pulmonary NTM disease in patients with rheumatoid arthritis who stop biologics have generally positive outcomes with NTM treatment, or stable NTM disease with no treatment, and deaths were related to underlying lung disease including pulmonary aspergillosis and interstitial lung disease.[43,47]

SOLID ORGAN TRANSPLANTS

Solid organ transplant recipients take a variety of immunosuppressive medications after transplantation. The most common maintenance drugs include calcineurin inhibitors (tacrolimus and cyclosporine), mammalian target of rapamycin (mTOR) inhibitor (sirolimus), prednisone, and others depending on the organ being transplanted. All data on NTM in transplants is found in case reports and institutional case series. To the authors' knowledge there are no population-based prevalence or incidence estimates to track trends or differences between transplant centers.

In a 2014 review of the literature including 293 solid organ transplant cases with NTM disease, lung transplant recipients had the most pulmonary NTM: 61% (61 of 100). Heart (11 of 45, 26%) and liver (5 of 16, 31%) transplant patients had similar amounts of pulmonary NTM, and kidney transplant patients had the lowest levels (22 of 132, 17%).[48] In a recent case-control study from a single institution, after excluding patients with NTM detected before transplant, lung transplant was the most important risk factor for NTM infection, accounting for 55.9% of cases (19 of 34).[49] All 4 NTM cases in liver transplant patients, 15 of 19 (78.9%) lung transplant patients, and the pancreas-kidney transplant patient had pleuropulmonary infection. Among solid organ transplant patients recently reviewed at 3 institutions, MAC and M abscessus each made up about 45% of the total 49 NTM infections.[49–51]

Diagnosis, Prevention, and Treatment

Treatment in transplant patients is complicated by drug interactions between rifamycin, macrolide, and aminoglycoside and calcineurin inhibitors (cyclosporine, sirolimus) and tacrolimus used after transplant, and should guide the selection of appropriate antibiotics.[52,53] There are several case reports of organ graft-versus-host disease in patients who decreased immunosuppressive medications, which needs to be balanced against the need for improved immune function for effective clearance or control of NTM disease.[48,53] Outcomes for renal transplant patients reported in a review of the literature are variable, with 41 (44%) of 94 cases considered resolved, 3 (3%) deaths (2 disseminated and 1 pulmonary), and 30 (32%) with complicated relapsed or long-term infection.[53] Outcomes for the 22 lung transplant patients were better, and included 7 (32%) who cleared NTM, 8 (36%) who showed improvement, 6 (27%) with no response or relapse, and 1 (5%) death from disseminated M abscessus.[53] More recent reports show very similar outcomes in 15 NTM cases in lung transplant patients at 2 institutions, with 9 (60%) clearing infection, 4 (27%) with persistent infection or recurring colonization, 1 (7%) unknown outcome, and 1 (7%) death from disseminated M abscessus.[50,51] To the authors' knowledge there are no published reports of deaths from NTM in heart transplant patients.

Lung transplant patients are at higher risk of NTM infection pretransplant, owing to the underlying condition that makes them eligible for transplant. Most transplant centers do not treat colonized patients, but should treat all pulmonary NTM disease in accordance with American Thoracic Society/Infectious Disease Society of America (ATS/IDSA) guidelines.[23,50] In the case of lung transplants in patients with cystic fibrosis, prior pulmonary M abscessus infection in patients is associated with mycobacterial infection after transplant. Based on evidence from one transplant center, M abscessus should not be considered a contraindication to lung transplant, and local control and clearance is possible if disease recurs.[54] Another institution's culture results before transplantation in 145 patients showed that 2 had NTM disease.[51] One was treated before and after single lung transplantation, and continued to test positive until his death from Aspergillosis pneumonia; the other was not treated and grew MAC 15 months after transplantation, but was not considered a case.

SOLID TUMORS AND HEMATOLOGIC MALIGNANCIES

Patients with cancer are at higher risk for NTM disease. Underlying cellular immunity impairment and immunosuppression from antineoplastic chemotherapy also contribute to the increased risk.[1,8,55] Patients with lung tumors are at increased risk of pulmonary NTM infection probably because of localized airway destruction or damage, and hematologic malignancies put patients at higher risk of both localized infections near the site of catheter placement and disseminated infections. Hairy cell leukemia is particularly associated with disseminated NTM disease, documented in the literature starting in the early 1980s.[6,7] A large institutional case series reported an incidence of 5% (9 of 186).[56] One estimate from Taiwan suggested that 1.2% of patients with hematologic malignancy developed NTM infections.[55]

HEMATOPOIETIC STEM CELL TRANSPLANTS

Hematopoietic stem cell transplants (HSCTs) are used to treat several hematologic malignancies, including leukemia, multiple myeloma, and others. The number of HSCTs has increased dramatically from 200 in 1980 to 20,000 in 2010.[57] The risks of NTM are higher before the transplant, owing to underlying immune cell abnormalities, and during the phase of immune reconstitution that follows induction immunosuppression and the HSCT. HSCTs are most frequently associated with catheter and blood infections, but 18% (17 of 97) were associated with pulmonary NTM in a 2014 review of NTM-infected HSCT patients.[53] Graft-versus-host disease was an important risk factor, present in 46% of NTM infections and corresponding with an increase in immunosuppressive medications.[53]

Overall, 26 of 93 (28%) were MAC/*M avium*, 23 (25%) were *M abscessus/M chelonae*, and 22 (24%) were *M haemophilum* infections. Most *M haemophilum* infections were associated with skin and catheter infection, but at least 5 pulmonary cases were reported among 19 cases in patients undergoing bone marrow transplant.[58–61] In a review of 571 allogeneic HSCTs, 16 NTM infections were identified, 3 (19%) of whom patients died of their NTM disease; this was one of the few studies to identify a high case fatality rate in immunosuppressed patients with NTM disease.[62] Nine of these infections were *M haemophilum*, 6 of which were associated with skin or catheter-related infections. In general, HSCT patients have a high rate of resolving infection after treatment and removal of catheters. However, death related to NTM occurred in 7 of 94 (7.5%) HSCT patients with pulmonary and disseminated NTM disease reported in the literature.[53] Treatment of *M haemophilum* and other rapidly growing mycobacterial disease should include prolonged therapy (see **Table 3**) and surgical removal of tissue as needed following catheter removal.[23]

PRIMARY IMMUNODEFICIENCY DISEASES

Primary immunodeficiency diseases include a large number of conditions associated with defects in antibody responses, and cellular and innate immunity.[63] A subset of these is associated with a documented or theoretic risk, and most are associated with the IL-12/IFN-γ axis.[63,64] Other conditions predisposing to NTM include chronic granulomatous disease, common variable immune deficiency, and hypogammaglobulinemia.[63] A recent study of conditions associated with death from NTM found that primary immunodeficiency was a comorbid cause of death in 2% of cases, more than for hematologic malignancies or HIV/AIDS.[16]

SUMMARY

Diseases and therapies that reduce cell-mediated immunity increase the risk of NTM disease. The broadening use of immunosuppressive drugs including anti-TNF biologics in the United States, and the expanding practice of stem cell and solid organ transplantation, places an increasing number of patients at risk for NTM disease.[38] With the exception of population-based studies of anti-TNF biologics and corticosteroids that report the risk of NTM at 8 to 50 times that of the general population, to date clinicians do not have sufficient understanding of the incidence of NTM disease in immunosuppressed populations.

Extrapulmonary NTM disease, including disseminated and skin and catheter-related disease, is more common in the immunosuppressed population. MAC remains the most common cause of NTM infection of all sites, but rapid growers including *M abscessus*, *M chelonae*, and *M fortuitum* are important causes of skin and catheter-related infections. With the exception of prophylaxis for AIDS patients with very low CD4+ counts, the prevention of NTM remains elusive. Management can be prolonged and difficult, and restoring immune function and removing catheters are essential alongside appropriate antibiotic treatment in accordance with current ATS/IDSA guidelines.[23]

REFERENCES

1. Feld R, Bodey GP, Groschel D. Mycobacteriosis in patients with malignant disease. Arch Intern Med 1976;136:67–70.
2. Havlik JA Jr, Horsburgh CR Jr, Metchock B, et al. Disseminated *Mycobacterium avium* complex infection: clinical identification and epidemiologic trends. J Infect Dis 1992;165:577–80.
3. Horsburgh CR Jr. *Mycobacterium avium* complex infection in the acquired immunodeficiency syndrome. N Engl J Med 1991;324:1332–8.
4. Lichtenstein IH, MacGregor RR. Mycobacterial infections in renal transplant recipients: report of five cases and review of the literature. Rev Infect Dis 1983;5:216–26.
5. Lloveras J, Peterson PK, Simmons RL, et al. Mycobacterial infections in renal transplant recipients. Seven cases and a review of the literature. Arch Intern Med 1982;142:888–92.
6. Gallo JH, Young GA, Forrest PR, et al. Disseminated atypical mycobacterial infection in hairy cell leukemia. Pathology 1983;15:241–5.
7. Weinstein RA, Golomb HM, Grumet G, et al. Hairy cell leukemia: association with disseminated atypical mycobacterial infection. Cancer 1981;48:380–3.
8. Rolston KV, Jones PG, Fainstein V, et al. Pulmonary disease caused by rapidly growing mycobacteria in patients with cancer. Chest 1985;87:503–6.
9. Cassidy PM, Hedberg K, Saulson A, et al. Nontuberculous mycobacterial disease prevalence and risk factors: a changing epidemiology. Clin Infect Dis 2009;49:e124–9.
10. Marras TK, Chedore P, Ying AM, et al. Isolation prevalence of pulmonary non-tuberculous mycobacteria in Ontario, 1997 2003. Thorax 2007;62:661–6.
11. Prevots DR, Shaw PA, Strickland D, et al. Nontuberculous mycobacterial lung disease prevalence at four integrated health care delivery systems. Am J Respir Crit Care Med 2010;182:970–6.

12. Winthrop KL, Varley CD, Ory J, et al. Pulmonary disease associated with nontuberculous mycobacteria, Oregon, USA. Emerg Infect Dis 2011;17:1760–1.

13. Andrejak C, Nielsen R, Thomsen VO, et al. Chronic respiratory disease, inhaled corticosteroids and risk of non-tuberculous mycobacteriosis. Thorax 2013; 68:256–62.

14. Henkle E, Hedberg K, Novosad S, et al. Incidence of nontuberculous mycobacterium disease in Oregon, 2007-2012. San Diego (CA): American Thoracic Society; 2014.

15. Winthrop KL, Baxter R, Liu L, et al. Mycobacterial diseases and antitumour necrosis factor therapy in USA. Ann Rheum Dis 2013;72:37–42.

16. Mirsaeidi M, Machado RF, Garcia JG, et al. Nontuberculous mycobacterial disease mortality in the United States, 1999-2010: a population-based comparative study. PLoS One 2014;9:e91879.

17. Ehlers S. Role of tumour necrosis factor (TNF) in host defence against tuberculosis: implications for immunotherapies targeting TNF. Ann Rheum Dis 2003; 62(Suppl 2):ii37–42.

18. Doherty T, Lynn M, Cavazza A, et al. *Mycobacterium haemophilum* as the initial presentation of a B-cell lymphoma in a liver transplant patient. Case Rep Rheumatol 2014;2014:742978.

19. Ducharlet K, Murphy C, Tan SJ, et al. Recurrent *Mycobacterium haemophilum* in a renal transplant recipient. Nephrology 2014;19(Suppl 1):14–7.

20. Lhuillier E, Brugiere O, Veziris N, et al. Relapsing *Mycobacterium genavense* infection as a cause of late death in a lung transplant recipient: case report and review of the literature. Exp Clin Transplant 2012;10:618–20.

21. Jones D, Havlir DV. Nontuberculous mycobacteria in the HIV infected patient. Clin Chest Med 2002;23: 665–74.

22. Winthrop KL, Baddley JW, Chen L, et al. Association between the initiation of anti-antitumor necrosis factor therapy and the risk of herpes zoster. JAMA 2013;309:887–95.

23. Griffith DE, Aksamit T, Brown-Elliott BA, et al. An official ATS/IDSA statement: diagnosis, treatment, and prevention of nontuberculous mycobacterial diseases. Am J Respir Crit Care Med 2007;175:367–416.

24. El Helou G, Hachem R, Viola GM, et al. Management of rapidly growing mycobacterial bacteremia in cancer patients. Clin Infect Dis 2013;56:843–6.

25. Winthrop KL, Chang E, Yamashita S, et al. Emerg Infect Dis. Emerg Infect Dis 2009;15:1556–61.

26. Kaplan JE, Hanson D, Dworkin MS, et al. Epidemiology of human immunodeficiency virus-associated opportunistic infections in the United States in the era of highly active antiretroviral therapy. Clin Infect Dis 2000;30(Suppl 1):S5–14.

27. Kaplan JE, Masur H, Holmes KK, USPHS, Infectious Disease Society of America. Guidelines for preventing opportunistic infections among HIV-infected persons—2002. Recommendations of the U.S. Public Health Service and the Infectious Diseases Society of America. MMWR Recomm Rep 2002;51:1–52.

28. Firth C, Capizzi J, Schafer S, et al. HIV/STD/TB Section, Public Health Division, Oregon Health Authority. Epidemiologic profile of HIV/AIDS in Oregon. 2013. Available at: http://public.health.oregon.gov/DiseasesConditions/CommunicableDisease/DiseaseSurveillanceData/HIVData/Documents/EpiProfile.pdf. Accessed August 18, 2014.

29. McCarthy KD, Cain KP, Winthrop KL, et al. Nontuberculous mycobacterial disease in patients with HIV in Southeast Asia. Am J Respir Crit Care Med 2012; 185:981–8.

30. Kaplan JE, Masur H, Holmes KK, et al. USPHS/IDSA guidelines for the prevention of opportunistic infections in persons infected with human immunodeficiency virus: an overview. USPHS/IDSA Prevention of Opportunistic Infections Working Group. Clin Infect Dis 1995;21(Suppl 1):S12–31.

31. Horsburgh CR Jr, Havlik JA, Ellis DA, et al. Survival of patients with acquired immune deficiency syndrome and disseminated *Mycobacterium avium* complex infection with and without antimycobacterial chemotherapy. Am Rev Respir Dis 1991;144:557–9.

32. Miguez-Burbano MJ, Flores M, Ashkin D, et al. Nontuberculous mycobacteria disease as a cause of hospitalization in HIV-infected subjects. Int J Infect Dis 2006;10:47–55.

33. Jick SS, Lieberman ES, Rahman MU, et al. Glucocorticoid use, other associated factors, and the risk of tuberculosis. Arthritis Rheum 2006;55:19–26.

34. Dirac MA, Horan KL, Doody DR, et al. Environment or host?: a case-control study of risk factors for *Mycobacterium avium* complex lung disease. Am J Respir Crit Care Med 2012;186:684–91.

35. Hojo M, Iikura M, Hirano S, et al. Increased risk of nontuberculous mycobacterial infection in asthmatic patients using long-term inhaled corticosteroid therapy. Respirology 2012;17:185–90.

36. Zumla A, James DG. Granulomatous infections: etiology and classification. Clin Infect Dis 1996;23: 146–58.

37. Gardam MA, Keystone EC, Menzies R, et al. Antitumour necrosis factor agents and tuberculosis risk: mechanisms of action and clinical management. Lancet Infect Dis 2003;3:148–55.

38. Winthrop KL, Chiller T. Preventing and treating biologic-associated opportunistic infections. Nat Rev Rheumatol 2009;5:405–10.

39. Novosad SA, Winthrop KL. Beyond tumor necrosis factor inhibition: the expanding pipeline of biologic therapies for inflammatory diseases and their associated infectious sequelae. Clin Infect Dis 2014;58: 1587–98.

40. Lee SK, Kim SY, Kim EY, et al. Mycobacterial infections in patients treated with tumor necrosis factor antagonists in South Korea. Lung 2013;191:565–71.

41. Yoo JW, Jo KW, Kang BH, et al. Mycobacterial diseases developed during anti-tumour necrosis factor-alpha therapy. Eur Respir J 2014;44(5):1289–95.

42. Cortet B, Flipo RM, Remy-Jardin M, et al. Use of high resolution computed tomography of the lungs in patients with rheumatoid arthritis. Ann Rheum Dis 1995;54:815–9.

43. Mori S, Tokuda H, Sakai F, et al. Radiological features and therapeutic responses of pulmonary nontuberculous mycobacterial disease in rheumatoid arthritis patients receiving biological agents: a retrospective multicenter study in Japan. Mod Rheumatol 2012;22:727–37.

44. Lutt JR, Pisculli ML, Weinblatt ME, et al. Severe nontuberculous mycobacterial infection in 2 patients receiving rituximab for refractory myositis. J Rheumatol 2008;35:1683–5.

45. Browne SK, Zaman R, Sampaio EP, et al. Anti-CD20 (rituximab) therapy for anti-IFN-gamma autoantibody-associated nontuberculous mycobacterial infection. Blood 2012;119:3933–9.

46. Czaja CA, Merkel PA, Chan ED, et al. Rituximab as successful adjunct treatment in a patient with disseminated nontuberculous mycobacterial infection due to acquired anti-interferon-gamma autoantibody. Clin Infect Dis 2014;58:e115–8.

47. Yamakawa H, Takayanagi N, Ishiguro T, et al. Clinical investigation of nontuberculous mycobacterial lung disease in Japanese patients with rheumatoid arthritis receiving biologic therapy. J Rheumatol 2013;40:1994–2000.

48. Knoll BM. Update on nontuberculous mycobacterial infections in solid organ and hematopoietic stem cell transplant recipients. Curr Infect Dis Rep 2014;16:421.

49. Longworth SA, Vinnard C, Lee I, et al. Risk factors for nontuberculous mycobacterial infections in solid organ transplant recipients: a case-control study. Transpl Infect Dis 2014;16:76–83.

50. Huang HC, Weigt SS, Derhovanessian A, et al. Nontuberculous mycobacterium infection after lung transplantation is associated with increased mortality. J Heart Lung Transplant 2011;30:790–8.

51. Knoll BM, Kappagoda S, Gill RR, et al. Non-tuberculous mycobacterial infection among lung transplant recipients: a 15-year cohort study. Transpl Infect Dis 2012;14:452–60.

52. Daley CL. Nontuberculous mycobacterial disease in transplant recipients: early diagnosis and treatment. Curr Opin Organ Transplant 2009;14:619–24.

53. Doucette K, Fishman JA. Nontuberculous mycobacterial infection in hematopoietic stem cell and solid organ transplant recipients. Clin Infect Dis 2004;38:1428–39.

54. Lobo LJ, Chang LC, Esther CR Jr, et al. Lung transplant outcomes in cystic fibrosis patients with pre-operative Mycobacterium abscessus respiratory infections. Clin Transplant 2013;27:523–9.

55. Chen CY, Sheng WH, Lai CC, et al. Mycobacterial infections in adult patients with hematological malignancy. Eur J Clin Microbiol Infect Dis 2012;31:1059–66.

56. Bennett C, Vardiman J, Golomb H. Disseminated atypical mycobacterial infection in patients with hairy cell leukemia. Am J Med 1986;80:891–6.

57. Pasquini MC, Wang Z. Current use and outcome of hematopoietic stem cell transplantation: CIBMTR summary slides. 2013. Available at: http://www.cibmtr.org. Accessed August 19, 2014.

58. Busam KJ, Kiehn TE, Salob SP, et al. Histologic reactions to cutaneous infections by Mycobacterium haemophilum. Am J Surg Pathol 1999;23:1379–85.

59. Kiehn TE, White M, Pursell KJ, et al. A cluster of four cases of Mycobacterium haemophilum infection. Eur J Clin Microbiol Infect Dis 1993;12:114–8.

60. Straus WL, Ostroff SM, Jernigan DB, et al. Clinical and epidemiologic characteristics of Mycobacterium haemophilum, an emerging pathogen in immunocompromised patients. Ann Intern Med 1994;120:118–25.

61. White MH, Papadopoulos EB, Small TN, et al. Mycobacterium haemophilum infections in bone marrow transplant recipients. Transplantation 1995;60:957–60.

62. Weinstock DM, Feinstein MB, Sepkowitz KA, et al. High rates of infection and colonization by nontuberculous mycobacteria after allogeneic hematopoietic stem cell transplantation. Bone Marrow Transplant 2003;31:1015–21.

63. Lee WI, Huang JL, Yeh KW, et al. Immune defects in active mycobacterial diseases in patients with primary immunodeficiency diseases (PIDs). J Formos Med Assoc 2011;110:750–8.

64. Sexton P, Harrison AC. Susceptibility to nontuberculous mycobacterial lung disease. Eur Respir J 2008;31:1322–33.

Nontuberculous Mycobacterial Infections in Cystic Fibrosis

Stacey L. Martiniano, MD[a],*, Jerry A. Nick, MD[b]

KEYWORDS

- Cystic fibrosis • Nontuberculous mycobacteria • Atypical mycobacteria
- *Mycobacterium avium* complex • *Mycobacterium abscessus*

KEY POINTS

- Patients with cystic fibrosis (CF) are at a very high risk of acquiring nontuberculous mycobacteria (NTM).
- NTM disease in CF patients is associated with bacterial coinfections, making diagnosis and treatment more challenging.
- *Mycobacterium avium* complex (MAC) and the *M abscessus* complex (MABSC) are the most frequently encountered NTM respiratory pathogens in CF patients.
- Diagnosis of NTM lung disease in CF patients generally follows American Thoracic Society (ATS) guidelines, with an emphasis on evaluating and treating all known comorbidities.
- Initial therapy for NTM respiratory pathogens in CF patients should be directed by published guidelines.
- Optimal management of patients with CF and NTM lung disease requires carefully considered treatment of both conditions.

INTRODUCTION

Over the past 2 decades, NTM have emerged as important pathogens in the setting of CF lung disease.[1] CF affects 1 in 3200 non-Hispanic whites in the United States due to autosomal recessive mutations in the CF transmembrane conductance regulator (CFTR) gene on chromosome 7. The impaired transport of sodium and chloride across epithelial surfaces, which occurs due to severely reduced CFTR function, results in viscous respiratory and gastrointestinal secretions leading to multiorgan disease. The principal cause of morbidity and mortality is obstruction of the small and medium-sized airways with dehydrated mucous plugs, resulting in bronchiectasis, chronic airway infections, and progression toward respiratory failure. Although historically considered a fatal disease of childhood, improvements in therapy have resulted in a steady increase in expected lifespan, with a current projected median survival of 37 years.[2] Replacement of pancreatic enzymes and supplementation with fat-soluble vitamins can compensate for malabsorption that arises from reduced exocrine pancreatic function.[3] A variety of airway clearance techniques combined with hydrating agents, mucolytics, and bronchodilators can assist mucociliary function and reduce bronchial obstruction.[4,5] Inhaled antibiotics targeting *Pseudomonas aeruginosa* have proved effective in both eradicating initial infection[6]

Disclosures: None.
[a] Department of Pediatrics, Children's Hospital Colorado, University of Colorado Denver School of Medicine, 13123 East 16th Avenue, B-395, Aurora, CO 80045, USA; [b] Department of Medicine, National Jewish Health, University of Colorado Denver, 1400 Jackson Street, Denver, CO 80206, USA
* Correspondence author.
E-mail address: Stacey.Martiniano@childrenscolorado.org

and in managing chronic infection.[5] More recently, the discovery of compounds that directly modulate the synthesis and/or function of CFTR protein have become available to a subgroup of CF patients based on their specific CFTR mutation.[7] As a result, the CF population is the oldest and healthiest in history.[2] But as the disease phenotype has changed in response to improved treatment, it seems that susceptibility to NTM has increased.[8–12]

Epidemiology

The ATS has identified the CF population as having both an especially high risk for NTM and posing unique challenges with regard to diagnosis and treatment.[13] Although the incidence of NTM disease in the general population of industrialized countries is approximately 1 in 100,000,[14] there is a 10,000-fold greater prevalence of these organisms in respiratory cultures from patients with CF. The reported prevalence of positive NTM cultures and/or NTM infection within various CF patient cohorts or at single centers varies dramatically,[15,16] but in the largest studies the overall the prevalence is 6% to 13%.[9,10,12,17–20] There is widespread agreement that the prevalence of NTM infection is increasing within the CF population,[1,8–12,21] as has been reported within the general population.[22,23] It is uncertain, however, to what extent improved culture techniques, increased physician awareness, and more frequent diagnosis of nonclassic forms of CF in adulthood may contribute to the apparent increase in NTM prevalence observed in this population.[24]

An overwhelming majority of NTM species recovered in CF samples in the United States are from either the MAC or the MABSC.[20] MAC has historically been the most common NTM isolated,[25–28] and in the largest US survey it was present in up to 72% of patients with NTM-positive sputum cultures.[9] The percentage of MABSC reported in CF patients with NTM-positive sputum cultures has ranged between 16% and 68%,[9,12,17,29] and it seems that the proportion of MABSC is increasing,[10,11,30] with some centers reporting a greater frequency than MAC. In part, this effect may be due to geographic factors, because MABSC seems especially prevalent in Europe,[1,12,17,29,30] and M simiae and MABSC are the most common species isolated in Israel.[31] Differences in relative prevalence of MAC and MABSC may also relate to the age of the cohorts studied, because MAC is more often associated with older CF patients and often diagnosed in adulthood, whereas MABSC is frequently seen in younger patients and those with more severe lung disease.[12,32] Less frequently isolated species include M kansasii[16,17,26,28] and M fortuitum.[8,17,27,33–35]

Risk Factors for Nontuberculous Mycobacteria in Cystic Fibrosis

Understanding of risk factors for NTM in CF patients is incomplete, because most reports have studied small cohorts from single centers or specific geographic areas, often leading to contradictory conclusions. The most worrisome trend from the largest population studies is that increased prevalence of NTM[9,11,18,27,30,31] and NTM disease[31,33] is strongly linked to older age and milder lung disease.[9] A high prevalence has been recorded in patients with an adult diagnosis,[25,36] which is typically associated with the nonclassic form of CF resulting from less severe mutations.[25,37] CFTR-related genotypes associated with partial CFTR function, such as D1152H, R75Q, and the 5T allele, have been specifically correlated with an increased frequency of NTM-positive cultures,[38,39] and in non-CF population, the presence of a single Q1352H allele has been linked to an increased prevalence of NTM disease.[40] The presence of Aspergillus fumigatus[11,31,41–43] has also been associated with increased risk for NTM, as has allergic bronchopulmonary aspergillosis (ABPA).[44,45] Coinfection with P aeruginosa has been associated with decreased prevalence of NTM.[9,28] Other studies, however, have reported the opposite conclusions, in particular that NTM is common in severe lung disease[18,31,33,46] and associated with higher rates of P aeurginosa coinfection.[31] These divergent findings may relate in part to differences in study methodology, because many reports have not distinguished between a positive NTM culture and the presence of NTM disease, and often culture data from MAC and MABSC are combined within both adult and pediatric populations.

Although increased survival may indirectly result in greater NTM prevalence through longer cumulative exposure,[47] a greater concern is the possibility that various medications and CF treatment strategies have contributed directly to the apparent increase in NTM prevalence. Although these reports are for the most part retrospective and their conclusions are not entirely consistent, they have served to heighten awareness of the potential for unforeseen consequences of many therapies in common use. In particular, administration of systemic steroids, often in the context of ABPA treatment, has been associated with increased prevalence of NTM[31,42,44,45] as well as high dose ibuprofen.[31] Other studies, however, have failed to see an increased in NTM-positive cultures with steroid use[18,31,48] or even an association with decreased NTM.[49] Azithromycin, an antibiotic with diverse anti-inflammatory properties, has also been associated with an increased prevalence of NTM,[31,50] although again other investigators have reported a decreased[51] or unchanged prevalence[48,52,53] in patients treated with the medication. Likewise, higher use of antipseudomonal antibiotics has been linked to increased NTM in some[16,31,54,55] but not all reports.[52] And, recently, the potential for patient-to-patient spread within CF centers has been described[56–59] with devastating consequences.[58]

PATIENT EVALUATION OVERVIEW—DIAGNOSIS OF NONTUBERCULOUS MYCOBACTERIAL DISEASE IN CYSTIC FIBROSIS
Laboratory Identification of Nontuberculous Mycobacteria in the Cystic Fibrosis Sputum

Historically, descriptions of NTM infection in CF patients were uncommon,[8,18,26,27,60] in part due to the lack of laboratory methodology specific to CF. Recovery of NTM from CF sputum samples was difficult due to coinfection with *P aeruginosa* and other microbes, which frequently overgrow the culture before the slower growing mycobacteria can be detected.[61–64] Development of effective sample decontamination protocols to remove conventional bacteria and fungi has allowed for culture-based detection of mycobacteria in CF samples.[65,66] Currently, the standard approach involves 2 steps[62] to avoid excessive decontamination, which can reduce NTM viability in samples.[67] Decontamination is first performed with *N*-acetyl-L-cysteine-NaOH, prior to mycobacterial culture.[62,65,66] Samples that remain contaminated can than be treated with oxalic acid, which may permit recovery of NTM, albeit with reduced sensitivity.[61,68] Alternatively, a second decontamination may be performed with 1% chlorhexidine, which may result in better recovery of mycobacteria but is less effective in eliminating residual sample contamination.[69]

Screening for Nontuberculous Mycobacteria in the Cystic Fibrosis Population

Frequently, nontuberculous mycobacteria are first detected in a CF sputum sample in the absence of clinical suspicion, as part of routine screening. It is generally accepted that surveillance for NTM in the CF population is worthwhile; however, the optimal frequency for such screening is not known. Balanced against the potential benefit of early detection of NTM disease is the risk of detecting NTM that is clinically not significant (discussed later). Certainly, the diagnosis can be missed in the absence of effective surveillance.[18] Small quantities of NTM from the environment may, however, intermittently be present in the CF airway but not result in NTM pulmonary disease,[9,49,70] raising

concern that too frequent screening may not effectively increase the detection of infection that warrants treatment. In the absence of clinical, microbiological, or radiologic suspicion of NTM infection, screening for NTM with an acid-fast bacilli (AFB) smear and culture on an annual basis has been recommended.[17,24,53,71]

Screening may also be considered in several other situations. A surveillance culture has been recommended prior to the initiation of chronic macrolide therapy to avoid exposing an unsuspected NTM infection to azithromycin as a single agent.[24,49] Attempted treatment of NTM with a single macrolide antibiotic has been implicated in increased development of resistance to the antibiotic,[72] which is a mainstay of treatment of both MAC and MABSC. Screening at a more frequent rate than once a year may also be considered in various patients deemed at higher risk for acquiring the infection or in which the infection could have more severe consequences. In particular, more frequent screening may be justified in older patients, those with advanced lung disease awaiting transplant, and those with previous NTM-positive cultures. Conversely, in small children and individuals not capable of producing a sputum sample, and with no recognized risk factors or clinical symptoms, NTM screening can be deferred.

Nearly all studies reporting prevalence of NTM in the CF population have used AFB smear and culture from sputum. Based on patient preference and the capacity of the CF center, either spontaneously expectorated sputum samples or sputum induced with hypertonic saline (HTS) can be used. No other methods have been validated for NTM detect in this setting, although NTM can on occasion be detected through laryngeal suction, oropharyngeal swabs, or gastric aspirate.[26,33,42,73,74] Skin testing for delayed-type hypersensitivity against NTM antigens does not seem sufficiently sensitive or specific to use for screening.[26,34,75] Going forward, it seems likely that culture-independent methods of NTM detection will be used. In particular, polymerase chain reaction techniques can be performed rapidly and are extremely sensitive and specific for the detection of NTM in sputum,[76–78] although not yet validated in the setting of CF. Likewise, serologic assays, such as IgG against mycobacterium antigen A60, for NTM surveillance seem promising[64,79] but currently lack validation in the CF population.

Cystic Fibrosis–Specific Diagnostic Considerations

Although technical aspects of recovering NTM from CF sputum samples have been improved, many aspects of the diagnosis of NTM disease in patients with CF remain uncertain. Unlike tuberculosis where a single positive culture can define disease, NTM species require repeated isolation prior to confirming the diagnosis of NTM lung disease. Because NTM are ubiquitous in the environment, the organism may appear transiently in a single sputum culture and apparently be eradicated by the host, with no clinical manifestations and negative cultures in subsequent samples.[49,70] Even for pathogenic NTM species isolated on more than one occasion, clinical sequelae can range from nondetectable to severe.[16,34,49,70,80,81] Thus, isolation of an NTM from a respiratory specimen is not synonymous with disease nor is it necessarily an indication to initiate treatment. Current ATS criteria for the diagnosis of NTM lung disease essentially calls for the presence of greater than 1 positive culture, in the setting of characteristic clinical symptoms and radiographic findings, and the exclusion of other diagnoses.[13] These guidelines have not been validated in any patient population and are particularly challenging in the setting of CF, where radiographic signs suggestive of NTM are common, and identical clinical symptoms can occur due to the near universal presence of coinfections with virulent pathogens, such as *P aeruginosa* and *Staphylococcus aureus*.[24] The central question for a patient who has cultured positive for a species of NTM on more than one occasion is whether this represents an indolent infection or actual NTM disease, which may benefit from treatment. Patients who are smear positive for NTM are more likely to have NTM disease[28,31] as are those who demonstrate progression by high-resolution CT of typical findings associated with NTM (**Fig. 1**).[49] Unexpectedly rapid

Pretreatment   Post-treatment

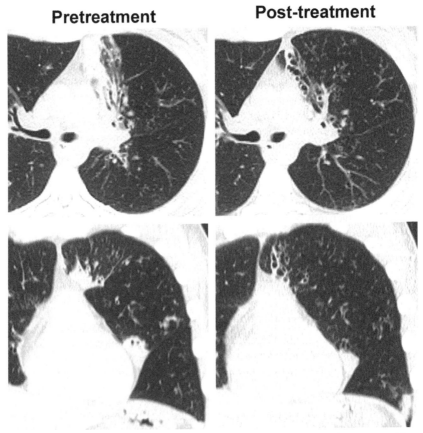

Fig. 1. Radiographic findings of NTM disease in CF. Axial and coronal CT images of a 25-year-old woman with CF diagnosed with NTM disease due to MAC as well as coinfection with *P aeruginosa*. Prior to treatment (*left panels*), typical CT features of NTM disease in CF are seen, including subsegmental parenchymal consolidation with atelectasis, nodules, and tree-and-bud opacities. After successful treatment (*right panels*), significant reduction in areas of consolidation and atelectasis are seen, although in some regions tree-and-bud opacities are more prominent, and a new area of consolidation is seen in the costophrenic angle. Together, these findings demonstrate that improvement in response to treatment of NTM is often accompanied by new abnormalities in other areas, and radiographic findings are not specific enough to distinguish between changes due to mycobacterial infection or other coinfection.

decline in forced expiratory volume in the first second of expiration (FEV$_1$) is frequently associated with NTM disease in patients with positive cultures for NTM.[33,82,83] In a recent retrospective study, a cohort of patients with NTM disease demonstrated a mean decline in FEV$_1$ for a year prior to initial recovery of NTM in their sputum, whereas patients with indolent infection or patients who apparently cleared the infection after a single positive culture demonstrated a stable FEV$_1$ for a year prior, and 3 years after, the initial positive culture.[70] Suggested criteria for the diagnosis of NTM disease in CF are outlined in **Box 1**.

PHARMACOLOGIC TREATMENT OPTIONS

There have been no completed trials evaluating antibiotic treatment regimens of NTM lung infection in people with CF.[84] Therefore, treatment of NTM pulmonary disease in CF should broadly be based on ATS and Infectious Disease Society of America (IDSA) guidelines that were developed

---

Box 1
Suggested criteria for the diagnosis of nontuberculous mycobacteria disease in the setting of cystic fibrosis; all 3 criteria should be met prior to treatment

1. Positive AFB cultures on at least 2 separate occasions, from either sputum or bronchoalveolar lavage.

2. Clinical symptoms consistent with NTM infection. At least one must be present, including
   - Unexplained loss in lung function
   - Increased respiratory symptoms (cough, sputum production, dyspnea, hemoptysis)
   - Constitutional symptoms, such as fever, night sweats, or weight loss
   - Progression of radiographic features consistent with NTM infection (cavitary disease, single or multiple nodules, tree-in-bud opacities, parenchymal consolidation)

3. Exclusion of other comorbidities common in CF, including adequate treatment of
   - Coinfections, such as P aeurginosa and S aureus
   - Airway clearance and reactive airways disease
   - Nutritional deficiencies
   - CF-related diabetes
   - Allergic bronchopulmonary aspergillosis
   - CF sinus disease

---

for the general population.[13] These treatment recommendations are reviewed in detail elsewhere in this issue by Kasperbauer and De Groote, and Philley and Griffith. Guidelines developed under the sponsorship of the United States Cystic Fibrosis Foundation (CFF) and the European Cystic Fibrosis Society specific to individuals with CF are under preparation, but these management recommendation are comprised solely of expert opinion and are not expected to differ substantially from that of the ATS/IDSA. Standard treatment regimens typically include at least 3 drugs directed against the specific NTM pathogen, in the oral, inhaled, and/or intravenous form.

Treatment Considerations Specific to Mycobacterium avium complex

Initial treatment of noncavitary NTM disease due to MAC uses a macrolide, rifampin, and ethambutol according to the guidelines for individuals with severe bronchiectatic disease.[13] Frequently, azithromycin is the macrolide chosen due to fewer interactions with rifampicin and the CYP3A enzyme system compared with clarithromycin[85] and a long history of use in CF lung disease. Azithromycin administration has recently been shown to reduce macrophage autophagy of M abscessus, suggesting that it has the potential to impair host defense independent of its antibiotic properties.[50] This potential detriment, however, has not been translated to patients with active NTM infection or to MAC. Additionally, chronic azithromycin therapy has been shown to have benefits in people with CF thought be due to immunomodulatory properties of the drug, in particular those patients with P aeruginosa.[86–89] Intermittent oral antibiotic therapy (ie, 3 times weekly) is not recommended in CF due to the presence of underlying lung disease and concerns of abnormal absorption of antimycobacterials and altered pharmacokinetics in CF.[90] In CF patients with MAC that is macrolide resistant, who are are systemically ill, who are AFB smear positive, or who have evidence of a cavitary lesion on chest imaging, a 1- to 3-month course of intravenous daily amikacin may be added at the beginning of the treatment course along with the standard 3 oral antibiotics. Patients within this category should generally be managed in collaboration with an expert in the treatment of NTM disease and CF.

Treatment of Mycobacterium abscessus complex

Treatment regimens for MABSC typically begin with an 8- to 12-week acute intensive phase of 3 antibiotics, including intravenous amikacin, cefoxitin, and/or imipenem, in addition to oral antibiotics. After intravenous therapy, patients typically continue on prolonged chronic suppressive therapy with oral and inhaled treatments with adjustments of therapy based on culture conversion as well as clinical and radiographic responses.[71] Changes to the drug regime are common, due to patient tolerance, side effects, and lack of efficacy. These patients should also be generally managed in collaboration with an expert in the treatment of NTM disease and CF.

Monitoring of Drug Toxicity and Clinical Response

Routine monitoring of drug toxicity is required, and a plan for monitoring should be set in place at the initiation of treatment. This is particularly important for patients on intravenous aminoglycosides. Patients with CF are commonly treated with aminoglycosides for other lung pathogens and, therefore, prone to auditory-vestibular toxicity and renal injury, making baseline and regular audiology evaluations and monitoring of renal function essential. Even among oral agents, the potential for drug-related side effects and toxicity is considerable, including bone marrow suppression and hepatitis. Of particular concern is change in visual acuity due to ethambutol. Patients are recommended to monitor their vision daily and the drug should be discontinued immediately at the first sign of vision disturbance. A monitoring schedule used within the Colorado CF Center is depicted in **Table 1**.

NONPHARMACOLOGIC AND COMBINATION TREATMENT OPTIONS

In addition to pharmacologic treatment of NTM infection, nonpharmacologic therapies for underlying CF lung disease that primarily target clearance of airway mucus obstruction are essential. CF lung disease is the result of a progressive cycle of mucus obstruction, chronic airway infections, and excessive inflammatory response.[91] All NTM treatment regimens need to be part of a comprehensive CF care plan that includes effective airway clearance, nutrition management, and treatment of CF comorbidities, such as sinus disease and CF-related diabetes. This care is most effectively delivered at a CF care center that uses a multidisciplinary approach, providing access to a respiratory therapist, dietitian, and social worker in addition to nurses and physicians experienced in CF care. CF care centers can be located at http://www.cff.org/LivingWithCF/CareCenterNetwork/CFFoundation-accreditedCareCenters/.

Airway Clearance

Airway clearance therapies (ACTs) are mechanical means of assisting patients in clearing secretions and mucus obstructing the airways. Routine ACT is recommended for all CF patients to maintain lung health.[4] No single form of ACT has been shown superior to others; therefore, the modality is chosen based on patient age, preference, and effectiveness in mobilizing airway secretions. The

Table 1
Example of a drug toxicity monitoring schedule for CF patients under treatment with standard antibiotics for nontuberculous mycobacterial disease

	CBC (+ Platelets)	LFTs (+ Albumin + Bilirubin)	Creatinine	Hearing	Visual[a]	P/K[b]	Examination for Neuropathy
Amikacin (intravenous)			Weekly	Monthly		After 1 wk	
Amikacin (inhaled)				Every 3 mo			
Cefoxitin	Monthly	Monthly	Monthly				
Macrolides	Monthly	Monthly		Every 3 mo			
Ethambutol	Monthly	Monthly	Monthly		Daily		Every 3 mo
Imipenem	Monthly	Monthly					
Rifampin	Monthly	Monthly	Monthly				
Tigecycline	Monthly	Monthly	Monthly				Every 3 mo
Clofazimine		Monthly	Monthly				
Linezolid	Monthly				Daily		Every 3 mo

Schedule of monitoring based on standard recommendations for each drug and consensus opinion, which should be modified for the individual patient based on pre-existing co-morbidities and underlying disease.
[a] Visual changes, including blurred vision, eye pain, red-green color blindness, or any loss of vision.
[b] Pharmacokinetic testing.

most commonly used forms of airway clearance include chest physiotherapy or percussion and postural drainage, positive expiratory pressure (PEP) or oscillatory PEP, and high-frequency chest compression with a vest device. To optimize mucus clearance, patients perform forced exhalation huff coughs in coordination with ACT to clear mucus. The method and frequency of airway clearance should be reviewed at every clinical visit during treatment of NTM.

Airway Surface Liquid and Mucus Alteration Treatments

The airway surface liquid is dehydrated in CF due to defective chloride transport by the CFTR protein, which impairs mucociliary clearance. HTS inhalation is a treatment that theoretically helps hydrate the airways in CF, accelerate mucus clearance, and improve lung function.[92,93] Typically HTS is preceded by administration of a bronchodilator to help prevent bronchospasm, a typical side effect of the treatment. Similarly, inhaled dry-powder mannitol (Bronchitol) is an osmotic agent available in the United Kingdom believed to increase surface liquid in the airways.[94] Recombinant human deoxyribonuclease or dornase alfa (Pulmozyme) is a nebulized medication designed to degrade extracellular DNA that accumulates within the CF mucus, thereby reducing mucus viscosity and promoting clearance of secretions.[95] These inhaled treatments are typically used in conjunction with ACT and help promote mucociliary clearance.

Prevention of Patient Transmission of Nontuberculous Mycobacteria in Cystic Fibrosis

Historically, infections with NTM have been thought to be from environmental exposure without evidence of patient-to-patient spread by pulse-field gel electrophoresis (PFGE).[17,96] Recently, there have been 2 reports of local outbreaks of *M abscessus* subsp *massiliense*. Five patients who had overlapping clinical encounters at the University of Washington Cystic Fibrosis Center were found to have identical isolates of *M abscessus* subsp *massiliense* by PFGE and repetitive unit sequence–based polymerase chain reaction pattern.[58] In the United Kingdom, another group used whole-genome sequencing as well as analysis of antibiotic resistance patterns to identify 2 clustered outbreaks of *M abscessus* subsp *massiliense*.[57] Although the exact transmission route was not established by epidemiologic analysis, both groups suspected indirect person-to-person spread within the clinic and hospital setting. There have been no reports to date with

evidence of patient transmission of MAC. Based on these recent outbreak reports and reports regarding other CF pathogens, the CFF recommends that all health care personnel implement contact precautions (eg, wear a gown and gloves) when caring for all people with CF, regardless of respiratory culture results, in both ambulatory and inpatient settings.[97] Additionally, they recommend that molecular typing of all NTM isolates be performed if there is a suspected patient-to-patient transmission event.[23]

SURGICAL TREATMENT OPTIONS

As discussed in depth by Mitchell elsewhere in this issue, surgical resection (pneumonectomy, lobectomy, or segmentectomy) may be a consideration as adjuvant therapy to medical treatment of NTM pulmonary disease. Generally, these recommendations are for non-CF patients with a localized focus of infection or cavitary pulmonary disease who have failed one or more courses of aggressive antibiotic therapy under the care of experienced physicians. In patients with CF, often there is a lobe with a greater burden of disease at a given point in time; however, disease is generally diffuse and bronchiectasis eventually involves all lobes. It is difficult to identify, with certainty, a focus of NTM infection in the setting of coinfection with typical CF pathogens, such as *P aeruginosa* and *S aureus*, and CF patients with a history of NTM are at high risk of acquiring a second NTM in their lifetime.[70] Finally, postoperative recovery may be slow in patients with CF, because airway clearance is limited by chest tubes and discomfort. For these reasons, surgical resection is rarely recommended. In rare circumstances, a CF patient with NTM disease may be identified who is a good candidate to benefit from lung resection but only in combination with intensive pre- and postoperative medical treatment and in the hands of an experienced thoracic surgeon.[13]

TREATMENT RESISTANCE/COMPLICATIONS

Currently, treatment success is generally defined by eradication of NTM from the sputum for 12 months after the discontinuation of antimicrobial therapy.[13,98] Rates of successful eradication seem to vary dramatically based on NTM species and patterns of antibiotic resistance, as seen in prospective trials in the general population discussed elsewhere in this issue by Kasperbauer and De Groote, and Philley and Griffith. In a recent retrospective review of CF patients from Colorado, the rate of eradication in response to initial treatment of MABSC (subspecies not designated) was 45%, and response to treatment of MAC was 60%.[70] Although no aspect of NTM treatment has been studied sufficiently, the issue of treatment failure is particularly problematic in the context of CF. General considerations in the evaluation of treatment failure include antibiotic resistance, inadequate dosing of the antibiotics, suboptimal airway clearance, lack of adherence to the prescribed medications, and the contribution of other comorbidities, including exacerbations of other chronic infections, chronic aspiration, and CF-related diabetes.

Therapeutic Drug Monitoring

Currently recommended dosages of antimycobacterials are based on pharmacokinetic and pharmacodynamic data from healthy volunteers and patients with tuberculosis. In one small case series, researchers demonstrated that serum levels of oral agents for the treatment of NTM are usually far below the target range in CF patients and in one case where treatment was failing, increasing the dose to achieve therapeutic levels was associated with eradication of the organism.[90] Even in patients with non-CF NTM disease, another series reported 48% of patients had low serum concentrations of ethambutol, 56% for clarithromycin, and 35% for azithromyin, despite using ATS/IDSA recommended doses.[85] Based on these studies and others, it seems that the dosing of patients with both CF and non-CF NTM disease may in some cases be subtherapeutic, possibly contributing to poor response to treatment.[90] Challenges to optimal dosing of CF patients include malabsorption of drug, impaired gastric motility, larger volume of distribution, increased metabolic rate, and potentially increased elimination.[99–101] In addition, drug-drug interactions may occur among various medications used to treat NTM, in particular, rifampin may increase the metabolism of macrolides and moxifloxacin.[85,102] Currently, it is standard practice to monitor amikacin serum levels when administered intravenously. Sufficient evidence is not available to recommend routine drug monitoring in all CF patients, but it should be considered in the setting of treatment failure.[103] In all CF patients, it must be emphasized that currently available antibiotics have significant limitation in achieving bacteriostatic concentrations within mucous plugs lodged in the airway[104]; thus, intensive airway clearance is an essential component of treatment (discussed previously).

Susceptibility Testing

Antimicrobial resistance may also contribute to treatment failure. To date, only the presence of

resistance to macrolides has been show to correlate with worse clinical outcomes.[13] Published guidelines by the Clinical and Laboratory Standards Institute have provided breakpoint concentrations to interpret minimum inhibitory concentrations as "susceptible" to a specific antibiotic, but these values are not validated in the CF airway. For these reasons, extensive antimicrobial testing is not generally recommended. In individual patients who are failing treatment despite therapeutic drug levels, susceptibility testing may be of value.[105] If not locally available, expanded drug susceptibility testing can be performed by sending the isolate to National Jewish Health in Denver, Colorado: http://www.nationaljewish.org/professionals/clinical-services/diagnostics/adx/about-us/diagnostic-lab-expertise/mycobacteriology/ast-ntm-aerobic-actinomycetes.

Clinical Response Without Eradication

To date, reports of therapeutic response to the treatment of NTM disease in both CF and non-CF patient cohorts have focused on rates of eradication of the organism.[13] Although this is certainly a primary goal of any initial treatment of NTM, it must be recognized that in the setting of CF lung disease, eradication often may not be achieved. Within individual patients, other clinical benefit may be appreciated from treatment of NTM disease, including improvement (or reduced decline) in FEV_1 and respiratory symptoms, reduced frequency of pulmonary exacerbations, resolution of systemic symptoms, and improvement in body mass index and in radiographic findings. Just as suppression of chronic P aeruginosa infection can achieve significant clinical benefits without eradication of the organisms,[5] a similar response to treatment may be seen in a case-by-case basis in CF patients with NTM disease. Guidance for suppressive treatment regimes of NTM are not available but may use the same drug combinations used for attempted eradication of the organism, based largely on the ability of patients to tolerate a specific combination of antibiotics. Particular emphasis must be placed on monitoring for drug toxicity. It seems reasonable that patients may be cycled on and off suppressive antibiotic combinations, with the duration of the treatment phase tailored to clinical response and the patient's ability to tolerate the therapy.

Lung Transplant in Cystic Fibrosis and Nontuberculous Mycobacteria

Bilateral lung transplant is an option considered by patients with CF who develop severe bronchiectasis and end-stage lung disease, generally described as an FEV_1 consistently below 30%

predicted, a rapid decline in FEV_1, or presence of increased frequency or severity of pulmonary exacerbations.[106] In 2006, the International Society for Heart and Lung Transplantation included colonization with highly resistant or highly virulent bacteria, fungi, or mycobacteria in the list of relative contraindications for lung transplant.[107] NTM-positive cultures and NTM pulmonary disease have been reported at a higher prevalence in CF patients referred for lung transplant compared with non-CF patients.[46] Case reports of death due to disseminated *M abscessus* post–lung transplant in adult and pediatric CF patients have been described in people with pretransplant infection,[108–110] although several patients have been described in which preexisting NTM was not detected but then was a source of post-transplant morbidity and mortality.[109,111,112] Chalermskulrat and colleagues[46] retrospectively analyzed their experience at the lung transplant center at University of North Carolina and described a 19.7% prevalence rate of NTM isolated from respiratory cultures from CF patients referred for transplant. Post-transplant, NTM disease prevalence was low but caused significant morbidity although no increase in mortality. More recently, a group from Denmark reviewed the 52 CF patients who underwent lung transplant at their center, describing a 21% prevalence of NTM-positive cultures pretransplant and a 17% prevalence of pretransplant NTM pulmonary disease. With perioperative medical treatment, 67% of their patients were alive at follow-up and no deaths had been attributed to NTM infection; however, morbidity, including wound infections, was described. Wound infections from *M abscessus* post-transplant have also been reported from Sweden in CF patients with pretransplant *M abscessus*.[112] Investigators from these studies have concluded that infection with NTM, even *M abscessus*, should not be an absolute contraindication to lung transplant, although morbidity is to be expected. Consensus opinion is that aggressive and prolonged courses of multiple antimycobacterial agents before transplant, perioperatively, and post-transplant are critical to improving outcomes in these patients.[109,113] At this time, the decision to proceed with lung transplant in patients with active MABSC disease is made individually by each US transplant program, with a majority declining to perform the transplant under this circumstance.

EVALUATION OF OUTCOME AND LONG-TERM RECOMMENDATIONS

For people with CF and positive NTM cultures or NTM pulmonary disease, clinical outcomes are not well reported in the literature. The capacity of NTM to accelerate progression of CF lung disease is reported; however, some reports have shown no clinical impact,[16] and others have shown groups of patients with transient sputum positivity only or apparent indolent infection.[18,59,64,70,80] In a longitudinal analysis of patients identified with NTM from the prospective US multicenter prevalence study, only 22 cases of NTM disease were identified, and the trend toward worsening lung function did not reach significance over the 15 months of follow-up.[49] In a large retrospective review with a mean of 6 years of follow-up, 38 cases of chronic NTM infection, defined by greater than or equal to 3 cultures, demonstrated greater decline in FEV_1 than a cohort without NTM, including a subset of 22 cases of chronic *M abscessus* infection but not in the subset without *M abscessus*.[11] Another large, longitudinal retrospective study demonstrated that by distinguishing patients who meet ATS criteria for NTM disease, the contribution of NTM to progression of CF lung disease is apparent within 3 years after the initial culture, irrespective of the type of NTM.[70] This decline in FEV_1 was seen even in the year preceding the date of the first positive NTM culture.

After a person with CF has been identified as having a positive NTM culture, close surveillance is warranted, with repeat sputum cultures obtained regularly.[13] Additionally, people with CF with clinical decline or radiographic progression of lung disease that is unresponsive to treatment of typical CF pathogens should be evaluated for NTM, in particular, patients previously infected with an NTM or treated for NTM pulmonary disease, because the presence of a second NTM is a common occurrence. In patients from the Colorado CF Center, MAC was typically the first identified NTM, but a subsequent positive culture for *M abscessus* was common, whereas subjects who first cultured *M abscessus* also had a high rate of secondary positive cultures for MAC.[70] Together, a remarkable 26% of subjects were identified, with a second NTM species at 5 years and 36% at 10 years (**Fig. 2**). Since the authors' initial publication, our experience is that this multiple NTM infection phenomenon occurs at an even higher rate (Stacey L. Martiniano and Jerry A. Nick, 2014, unpublished data). Many previous trials have also anecdotally noted the presence of individuals with more than one species of NTM recovered from their sputum.[9–11,27,30–32,59] These findings support the need for lifelong strategies for NTM surveillance and management in CF patients who present with a positive NTM culture.

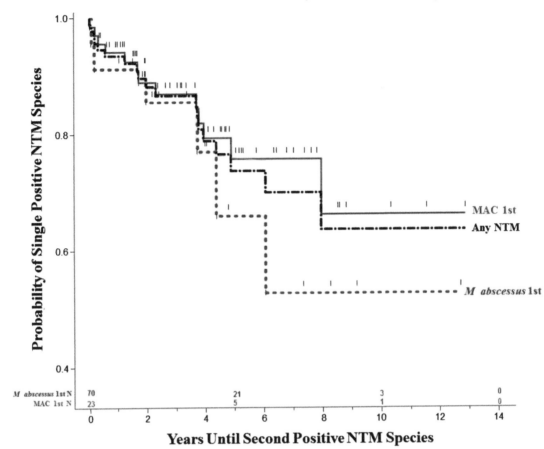

Fig. 2. Probability of detecting a second NTM species after culturing a first NTM. Following an initial positive culture, 24% of subjects with MAC initially grew a second NTM species during 5 years of follow-up, while 34% with *M abscessus* first grew a second NTM species at 5 years. Overall, 26% of subjects grew a second NTM species at 5 years and 36% at 10 years. Kaplan-Meier analysis, separated by initial positive NTM culture species. Reprinted with permission of the American Thoracic Society. Copyright © 2014 American Thoracic Society. Martiniano SL, Sontag MK, Daley CL, et al. Clinical significance of a first positive nontuberculous mycobacteria culture in cystic fibrosis. Ann Am Thorac Soc 2014;11:41. Official Journal of the American Thoracic Society.

SUMMARY/DISCUSSION

Based on current trends, it seems likely that NTM will continue to increase in prevalence within the CF population. The steady improvement in survival achieved over the past 2 decades may be accelerated as CFTR modulators become more widely available. These agents partially restore CFTR function to levels similar to nonclassic CF patients with 1 or more naturally occurring partial function CFTR mutations.[114] Thus, a greater proportion of the CF population will resemble the phenotype best suited to MAC infection, which correlated with less severe CFTR mutations[25,38,39] and greater age.[9,18,27,31,33] Independently, it seems that the prevalence of MABSC is increasing,[10,11,30]

in some cases apparently due to patient-to-patient transmission,[56–59] and that children and patients with more severe pulmonary disease are at risk.[12,32] When these trends are viewed in the context of a global increase in NTM burden within the modern environment,[115–117] the need for evidence-based strategies toward NTM in the CF population is evident. Treatment presents a significant burden on both patient and provider,[118] requiring a prolonged multidrug regimen, often including several months of multiple continuous intravenous antibiotics. Treatment is frequently associated with drug toxicities and side effects, with no assurance of sustained sputum clearance of the pathogen. For CF patients, this treatment burden comes in addition to existing time- and cost-intensive regimens of medications and airway clearance. Because treatment may not be necessary in all cases, a CF-specific diagnostic criterion with both high sensitivity and specificity is a pressing need. Equally important is the need for validated markers of disease response, including treatment endpoints. A significant investment in NTM-related research will be required over the next decades to meet this challenge. The CF patient population, however, is uniquely served by the CFF Therapeutics Development Network, which has a long track record of success in developing new therapies and testing treatment strategies,[119] and this infrastructure may allow for much needed prospective trials in NTM disease.

ACKNOWLEDGMENTS

Support provided by the Cystic Fibrosis Foundation (NICK13A0), and the Rebecca Runyon Bryan Chair for Cystic Fibrosis.

REFERENCES

1. Qvist T, Pressler T, Hoiby N, et al. Shifting paradigms of nontuberculous mycobacteria in cystic fibrosis. Respir Res 2014;15:41.

2. Cystic Fibrosis Foundation Patient Registry. 2012 annual data report to the center directors. Bethesda (MD): Cystic Fibrosis Foundation; 2013.

3. Stallings VA, Stark LJ, Robinson KA, et al, Clinical Practice Guidelines on Growth and Nutrition Subcommittee, Ad Hoc Working Group. Evidence-based practice recommendations for nutrition-related management of children and adults with cystic fibrosis and pancreatic insufficiency: results of a systematic review. J Am Diet Assoc 2008;108:832–9.

4. Flume PA, Robinson KA, O'Sullivan BP, et al. Cystic fibrosis pulmonary guidelines: airway clearance therapies. Respir Care 2009;54:522–37.

5. Mogayzel PJ Jr, Naureckas ET, Robinson KA, et al, Pulmonary Clinical Practice Guidelines Committee. Cystic fibrosis pulmonary guidelines. Chronic medications for maintenance of lung health. Am J Respir Crit Care Med 2013;187:680–9.

6. Ratjen F, Munck A, Kho P, et al. Treatment of early pseudomonas aeruginosa infection in patients with cystic fibrosis: the elite trial. Thorax 2010;65:286–91.

7. Ong T, Ramsey BW. Modifying disease in cystic fibrosis: current and future therapies on the horizon. Curr Opin Pulm Med 2013;19:645–51.

8. Smith MJ, Efthimiou J, Hodson ME, et al. Mycobacterial isolations in young adults with cystic fibrosis. Thorax 1984;39:369–75.

9. Olivier KN, Weber DJ, Wallace RJ Jr, et al. Nontuberculous mycobacteria. I: multicenter prevalence study in cystic fibrosis. Am J Respir Crit Care Med 2003;167:828–34.

10. Roux AL, Catherinot E, Ripoll F, et al, Jean-Louis Herrmann for the OMA Group. Multicenter study of prevalence of nontuberculous mycobacteria in patients with cystic fibrosis in france. J Clin Microbiol 2009;47:4124–8.

11. Esther CR Jr, Esserman DA, Gilligan P, et al. Chronic mycobacterium abscessus infection and lung function decline in cystic fibrosis. J Cyst Fibros 2010;9:117–23.

12. Qvist T, Gilljam M, Jonsson B, et al, the Scandinavian Cystic Fibrosis Study Consortium (SCFSC). Epidemiology of nontuberculous mycobacteria among patients with cystic fibrosis in scandinavia. J Cyst Fibros 2014;14:S1569–1993.

13. Griffith DE, Aksamit T, Brown-Elliott BA, et al. An official ats/idsa statement: diagnosis, treatment, and prevention of nontuberculous mycobacterial diseases. Am J Respir Crit Care Med 2007;175:367–416.

14. Hsorsburgh CR. Epidemiology of mycobacterium avium complex. In: Korvick JA, Benson CA, editors. Mycobacterium avium complex infection: progress in research and treatment. New York: Marcel Dekker; 1996. p. 1–22.

15. Andre E, Degraux J, Simon A, et al. Absence of nontuberculous mycobacteria recovery in sputum of cystic fibrosis patients despite adequate decontamination: a possible role of specific antimicrobial therapy used in our centre. Clin Microbiol Infect 2010;16:S33–4.

16. Torrens JK, Dawkins P, Conway SP, et al. Nontuberculous mycobacteria in cystic fibrosis. Thorax 1998;53:182–5.

17. Sermet-Gaudelus I, Le Bourgeois M, Pierre-Audigier C, et al. Mycobacterium abscessus and children with cystic fibrosis. Emerg Infect Dis 2003;9:1587–91.

18. Aitken ML, Burke W, McDonald G, et al. Nontuberculous mycobacterial disease in adult cystic fibrosis patients. Chest 1993;103:1096–9.

19. Valenza G, Tappe D, Turnwald D, et al. Prevalence and antimicrobial susceptibility of microorganisms isolated from sputa of patients with cystic fibrosis. J Cyst Fibros 2008;7:123–7.

20. Adjemian J, Olivier KN, Prevots DR. Nontuberculous mycobacteria among cystic fibrosis patients in the united states: screening practices and environmental risk. Am J Respir Crit Care Med 2014;190(5):581–6.

21. Leung JM, Olivier KN. Nontuberculous mycobacteria: the changing epidemiology and treatment challenges in cystic fibrosis. Curr Opin Pulm Med 2013; 19:662–9.

22. Adjemian J, Olivier KN, Seitz AE, et al. Prevalence of nontuberculous mycobacterial lung disease in U.S. Medicare beneficiaries. Am J Respir Crit Care Med 2012;185:881–6.

23. Prevots DR, Shaw PA, Strickland D, et al. Nontuberculous mycobacterial lung disease prevalence at four integrated health care delivery systems. Am J Respir Crit Care Med 2010;182:970–6.

24. Leung JM, Olivier KN. Nontuberculous mycobacteria in patients with cystic fibrosis. Semin Respir Crit Care Med 2013;34:124–34.

25. Rodman DM, Polis JM, Heltshe SL, et al. Late diagnosis defines a unique population of long-term survivors of cystic fibrosis. Am J Respir Crit Care Med 2005;171:621–6.

26. Hjelte L, Petrini B, Kallenius G, et al. Prospective study of mycobacterial infections in patients with cystic fibrosis. Thorax 1990;45:397–400.

27. Kilby JM, Gilligan PH, Yankaskas JR, et al. Nontuberculous mycobacteria in adult patients with cystic fibrosis. Chest 1992;102:70–5.

28. Esther CR Jr, Henry MM, Molina PL, et al. Nontuberculous mycobacterial infection in young children with cystic fibrosis. Pediatr Pulmonol 2005; 40:39–44.

29. Seddon P, Fidler K, Raman S, et al. Prevalence of nontuberculous mycobacteria in cystic fibrosis clinics, united kingdom, 2009. Emerg Infect Dis 2013;19:1128–30.

30. Pierre-Audigier C, Ferroni A, Sermet-Gaudelus I, et al. Age-related prevalence and distribution of nontuberculous mycobacterial species among patients with cystic fibrosis. J Clin Microbiol 2005;43: 3467–70.

31. Levy I, Grisaru-Soen G, Lerner-Geva L, et al. Multicenter cross-sectional study of nontuberculous mycobacterial infections among cystic fibrosis patients, israel. Emerg Infect Dis 2008;14:378–84.

32. Catherinot E, Roux AL, Vibet MA, et al. Mycobacterium avium and mycobacterium abscessus complex target distinct cystic fibrosis patient subpopulations. J Cyst Fibros 2013;12:74–80.

33. Fauroux B, Delaisi B, Clement A, et al. Mycobacterial lung disease in cystic fibrosis: a prospective study. Pediatr Infect Dis J 1997;16:354–8.

34. Hjelt K, Hojlyng N, Howitz P, et al. The role of mycobacteria other than tuberculosis (mott) in patients with cystic fibrosis. Scand J Infect Dis 1994;26: 569–76.

35. Aitken ML, Moss RB, Waltz DA, et al. A phase I study of aerosolized administration of tgAAVCF to cystic fibrosis subjects with mild lung disease. Hum Gene Ther 2001;12:1907–16.

36. Keating CL, Liu X, Dimango EA. Classic respiratory disease but atypical diagnostic testing distinguishes adult presentation of cystic fibrosis. Chest 2010;137:1157–63.

37. Nick JA, Chacon CS, Brayshaw SJ, et al. Effects of gender and age at diagnosis on disease progression in long-term survivors of cystic fibrosis. Am J Respir Crit Care Med 2010;182:614–26.

38. Ziedalski TM, Kao PN, Henig NR, et al. Prospective analysis of cystic fibrosis transmembrane regulator mutations in adults with bronchiectasis or pulmonary nontuberculous mycobacterial infection. Chest 2006;130:995–1002.

39. Kim JS, Tanaka N, Newell JD, et al. Nontuberculous mycobacterial infection: CT scan findings, genotype, and treatment responsiveness. Chest 2005; 128:3863–9.

40. Jang MA, Kim SY, Jeong BH, et al. Association of CFTR gene variants with nontuberculous mycobacterial lung disease in a korean population with a low prevalence of cystic fibrosis. J Hum Genet 2013; 58:298–303.

41. Burgel P, Morand P, Audureau E, et al. Azithromycin and the risk of nontuberculous mycobacteria in adults with cystic fibrosis. Pediatr Pulmonol 2011;46:328.

42. Ager S, O'Brien C, Spencer DA, et al. A retrospective review of non-tuberculous mycobacteria in paediatric cystic fibrosis patients at a regional centre. J Cyst Fibros 2011;10:S36.

43. Paugam A, Baixench MT, Demazes-Dufeu N, et al. Characteristics and consequences of airway colonization by filamentous fungi in 201 adult patients with cystic fibrosis in france. Med Mycol 2010; 48(Suppl 1):S32–6.

44. Mussaffi H, Rivlin J, Shalit I, et al. Nontuberculous mycobacteria in cystic fibrosis associated with allergic bronchopulmonary aspergillosis and steroid therapy. Eur Respir J 2005;25:324–8.

45. Evans JT, Ratnaraja N, Gardiner S, et al. Mycobacterium abscessus in cystic fibrosis: what does it all mean? Clin Microbiol Infect 2011;17:S602.

46. Chalermskulrat W, Sood N, Neuringer IP, et al. Nontuberculous mycobacteria in end stage cystic fibrosis: implications for lung transplantation. Thorax 2006;61:507–13.

47. Falkinham JO 3rd. Surrounded by mycobacteria: nontuberculous mycobacteria in the human environment. J Appl Microbiol 2009;107:356–67.

48. Giron RM, Maiz L, Barrio I, et al. nontuberculous mycobacterial infection in patients with cystic fibrosis: a multicenter prevalence study. Arch Bronconeumol 2008;44:679–84 [in Spanish].

49. Olivier KN, Weber DJ, Lee JH, et al. Nontuberculous mycobacteria. II: nested-cohort study of impact on cystic fibrosis lung disease. Am J Respir Crit Care Med 2003;167:835–40.

50. Renna M, Schaffner C, Brown K, et al. Azithromycin blocks autophagy and may predispose cystic fibrosis patients to mycobacterial infection. J Clin Invest 2011;121:3554–63.

51. Binder AM, Adjemian J, Olivier KN, et al. Epidemiology of nontuberculous mycobacterial infections and associated chronic macrolide use among persons with cystic fibrosis. Am J Respir Crit Care Med 2013;188:807–12.

52. Catherinot E, Roux AL, Vibet MA, et al, OMA Group. Inhaled therapies, azithromycin and mycobacterium abscessus in cystic fibrosis patients. Eur Respir J 2013;41:1101–6.

53. Radhakrishnan DK, Yau Y, Corey M, et al. Nontuberculous mycobacteria in children with cystic fibrosis: isolation, prevalence, and predictors. Pediatr Pulmonol 2009;44:1100–6.

54. Bowker JL, Thomas MF, O'Brien CJ. Antibiotic usage as a risk factor for non-tuberculous mycobacterium infection in children with cystic fibrosis. Thorax 2013;68:A111–2.

55. MacNeil SJ, Vamvakas G, Rosenthal M. NTM: lessons from the UK CF registry. J Cyst Fibros 2014; 13:S71.

56. Harris KA, Kenna DT, Blauwendraat C, et al. Molecular fingerprinting of mycobacterium abscessus strains in a cohort of pediatric cystic fibrosis patients. J Clin Microbiol 2012;50:1758–61.

57. Bryant JM, Grogono DM, Greaves D, et al. Whole-genome sequencing to identify transmission of mycobacterium abscessus between patients with cystic fibrosis: a retrospective cohort study. Lancet 2013;381:1551–60.

58. Aitken ML, Limaye A, Pottinger P, et al. Respiratory outbreak of mycobacterium abscessus subspecies massiliense in a lung transplant and cystic fibrosis center. Am J Respir Crit Care Med 2012;185:231–2.

59. Jonsson BE, Gilljam M, Lindblad A, et al. Molecular epidemiology of mycobacterium abscessus, with focus on cystic fibrosis. J Clin Microbiol 2007;45: 1497–504.

60. Boxerbaum B. Isolation of rapidly growing mycobacteria in patients with cystic fibrosis. J Pediatr 1980;96:689–91.

61. Whittier S, Olivier K, Gilligan P, et al. Proficiency testing of clinical microbiology laboratories using modified decontamination procedures for detection of nontuberculous mycobacteria in sputum samples from cystic fibrosis patients. The nontuberculous mycobacteria in cystic fibrosis study group. J Clin Microbiol 1997;35:2706–8.

62. Bange FC, Bottger EC. Improved decontamination method for recovering mycobacteria from patients with cystic fibrosis. Eur J Clin Microbiol Infect Dis 2002;21:546–8.

63. Whittier S, Hopfer RL, Knowles MR, et al. Improved recovery of mycobacteria from respiratory secretions of patients with cystic fibrosis. J Clin Microbiol 1993;31:861–4.

64. Oliver A, Maiz L, Canton R, et al. Nontuberculous mycobacteria in patients with cystic fibrosis. Clin Infect Dis 2001;32:1298–303.

65. Steingart KR, Ng V, Henry M, et al. Sputum processing methods to improve the sensitivity of smear microscopy for tuberculosis: a systematic review. Lancet Infect Dis 2006;6:664–74.

66. Brown-Elliott BA, Griffith DE, Wallace RJ Jr. Diagnosis of nontuberculous mycobacterial infections. Clin Lab Med 2002;22:911–25, vi.

67. Buijtels PC, Petit PL. Comparison of naoh-n-acetyl cysteine and sulfuric acid decontamination methods for recovery of mycobacteria from clinical specimens. J Microbiol Methods 2005;62:83–8.

68. Bange FC, Kirschner P, Bottger EC. Recovery of mycobacteria from patients with cystic fibrosis. J Clin Microbiol 1999;37:3761–3.

69. Ferroni A, Vu-Thien H, Lanotte P, et al. Value of the chlorhexidine decontamination method for recovery of nontuberculous mycobacteria from sputum samples of patients with cystic fibrosis. J Clin Microbiol 2006;44:2237–9.

70. Martiniano SL, Sontag MK, Daley CL, et al. Clinical significance of a first positive nontuberculous mycobacteria culture in cystic fibrosis. Ann Am Thorac Soc 2014;11:36–44.

71. Ebert DL, Olivier KN. Nontuberculous mycobacteria in the setting of cystic fibrosis. Clin Chest Med 2002;23:655–63.

72. Doucet-Populaire F, Buriankova K, Weiser J, et al. Natural and acquired macrolide resistance in mycobacteria. Curr Drug Targets Infect Disord 2002;2: 355–70.

73. Verma N, Spencer D. Disseminated mycobacterium gordonae infection in a child with cystic fibrosis. Pediatr Pulmonol 2012;47:517–8.

74. Segal E, Diez GS, Prokopio E, et al. Nontuberculous mycobacteria in patients with cystic fibrosis. Medicina 1998;58:257–61 [in Spanish].

75. Mulherin D, Coffey MJ, Halloran DO, et al. Skin reactivity to atypical mycobacteria in cystic fibrosis. Respir Med 1990;84:273–6.

76. Ngan GJ, Ng LM, Jureen R, et al. Development of multiplex pcr assays based on the 16s-23s rrna internal transcribed spacer for the detection of clinically relevant nontuberculous mycobacteria. Lett Appl Microbiol 2011;52:546–54.

77. Leung KL, Yip CW, Cheung WF, et al. Development of a simple and low-cost real-time pcr method for the identification of commonly encountered mycobacteria in a high throughput laboratory. J Appl Microbiol 2009;107:1433–9.

78. Devine M, Moore JE, Xu J, et al. Detection of mycobacterial DNA from sputum of patients with cystic fibrosis. Ir J Med Sci 2004;173:96–8.

79. Ferroni A, Sermet-Gaudelus I, Le Bourgeois M, et al. Measurement of immunoglobulin g against mycobacterial antigen a60 in patients with cystic fibrosis and lung infection due to mycobacterium abscessus. Clin Infect Dis 2005;40:58–66.

80. Cullen AR, Cannon CL, Mark EJ, et al. Mycobacterium abscessus infection in cystic fibrosis. Colonization or infection? Am J Respir Crit Care Med 2000;161:641–5.

81. Catherinot E, Roux AL, Macheras E, et al. Acute respiratory failure involving an r variant of mycobacterium abscessus. J Clin Microbiol 2009;47:271–4.

82. Forslow U, Geborek A, Hjelte L, et al. Early chemotherapy for non-tuberculous mycobacterial infections in patients with cystic fibrosis. Acta Paediatr 2003;92:910–5.

83. Leitritz L, Griese M, Roggenkamp A, et al. Prospective study on nontuberculous mycobacteria in patients with and without cystic fibrosis. Med Microbiol Immunol 2004;193:209–17.

84. Waters V, Ratjen F. Antibiotic treatment for nontuberculous mycobacteria lung infection in people with cystic fibrosis. Cochrane Database Syst Rev 2012;(12):CD010004.

85. van Ingen J, Egelund EF, Levin A, et al. The pharmacokinetics and pharmacodynamics of pulmonary mycobacterium avium complex disease treatment. Am J Respir Crit Care Med 2012; 186(6):559–65.

86. Clement A, Tamalet A, Leroux E, et al. Long term effects of azithromycin in patients with cystic fibrosis: a double blind, placebo controlled trial. Thorax 2006;61:895–902.

87. Equi A, Balfour-Lynn IM, Bush A, et al. Long term azithromycin in children with cystic fibrosis: a randomised, placebo-controlled crossover trial. Lancet 2002;360:978–84.

88. Saiman L, Marshall BC, Mayer-Hamblett N, et al. Azithromycin in patients with cystic fibrosis chronically infected with pseudomonas aeruginosa: a randomized controlled trial. JAMA 2003;290: 1749–56.

89. Wolter J, Seeney S, Bell S, et al. Effect of long term treatment with azithromycin on disease parameters in cystic fibrosis: a randomised trial. Thorax 2002; 57:212–6.

90. Gilljam M, Berning SE, Peloquin CA, et al. Therapeutic drug monitoring in patients with cystic fibrosis and mycobacterial disease. Eur Respir J 1999;14:347–51.

91. Anselmo MA, Lands LC. Cystic fibrosis: overview. In: Taussig LM, Landau LI, editors. Pediatric respiratory medicine. 2nd edition. Philadelphia: Mosby Inc; 2008. p. 845–57.

92. Donaldson SH, Bennett WD, Zeman KL, et al. Mucus clearance and lung function in cystic fibrosis with hypertonic saline. N Engl J Med 2006;354:241–50.

93. Elkins MR, Robinson M, Rose BR, et al. A controlled trial of long-term inhaled hypertonic saline in patients with cystic fibrosis. N Engl J Med 2006;354:229–40.

94. Aitken ML, Bellon G, De Boeck K, et al. Long-term inhaled dry powder mannitol in cystic fibrosis: an international randomized study. Am J Respir Crit Care Med 2012;185:645–52.

95. Fuchs HJ, Borowitz DS, Christiansen DH, et al. Effect of aerosolized recombinant human dnase on exacerbations of respiratory symptoms and on pulmonary function in patients with cystic fibrosis. The pulmozyme study group. N Engl J Med 1994;331: 637–42.

96. Bange FC, Brown BA, Smaczny C, et al. Lack of transmission of mycobacterium abscessus among patients with cystic fibrosis attending a single clinic. Clin Infect Dis 2001;32:1648–50.

97. Saiman L, Siegel JD, LiPuma JJ, et al. Infection prevention and control guideline for cystic fibrosis: 2013 update. Infect Control Hosp Epidemiol 2014; 35:S1–67.

98. Jarand J, Levin A, Zhang L, et al. Clinical and microbiologic outcomes in patients receiving treatment for mycobacterium abscessus pulmonary disease. Clin Infect Dis 2011;52:565–71.

99. Kearns GL, Trang JM. Introduction to pharmacokinetics: aminoglycosides in cystic fibrosis as a prototype. J Pediatr 1986;108:847–53.

100. de Groot R, Smith AL. Antibiotic pharmacokinetics in cystic fibrosis. Differences and clinical significance. Clin Pharmacokinet 1987;13:228–53.

101. Rey E, Treluyer JM, Pons G. Drug disposition in cystic fibrosis. Clin Pharmacokinet 1998;35: 313–29.

102. Wallace RJ Jr, Brown BA, Griffith DE, et al. Reduced serum levels of clarithromycin in patients treated with multidrug regimens including rifampin or rifabutin for mycobacterium avium-m. Intracellulare infection. J Infect Dis 1995;171:747–50.

103. Peloquin CA. Therapeutic drug monitoring in the treatment of tuberculosis. Drugs 2002;62: 2169–83.

104. Moriarty TF, McElnay JC, Elborn JS, et al. Sputum antibiotic concentrations: implications for treatment of cystic fibrosis lung infection. Pediatr Pulmonol 2007;42:1008–17.

105. Huang YC, Liu MF, Shen GH, et al. Clinical outcome of mycobacterium abscessus infection and antimicrobial susceptibility testing. J Microbiol Immunol Infect 2010;43:401–6.

106. Braun AT, Merlo CA. Cystic fibrosis lung transplantation. Curr Opin Pulm Med 2011;17:467–72.

107. Orens JB, Estenne M, Arcasoy S, et al. International guidelines for the selection of lung transplant candidates: 2006 update–a consensus report from the pulmonary scientific council of the international society for heart and lung transplantation. J Heart Lung Transpl 2006;25:745–55.

108. Taylor JL, Palmer SM. Mycobacterium abscessus chest wall and pulmonary infection in a cystic fibrosis lung transplant recipient. J Heart Lung Transpl 2006;25:985–8.

109. Zaidi S, Elidemir O, Heinle JS, et al. Mycobacterium abscessus in cystic fibrosis lung transplant

recipients: report of 2 cases and risk for recurrence. Transpl Infect Dis 2009;11:243–8.

110. Sanguinetti M, Ardito F, Fiscarelli E, et al. Fatal pulmonary infection due to multidrug-resistant mycobacterium abscessus in a patient with cystic fibrosis. J Clin Microbiol 2001;39:816–9.

111. Flume PA, Egan TM, Paradowski LJ, et al. Infectious complications of lung transplantation. Impact of cystic fibrosis. Am J Respir Crit Care Med 1994; 149:1601–7.

112. Gilljam M, Schersten H, Silverborn M, et al. Lung transplantation in patients with cystic fibrosis and mycobacterium abscessus infection. J Cyst Fibros 2010;9:272–6.

113. Watkins RR, Lemonovich TL. Evaluation of infections in the lung transplant patient. Curr Opin Infect Dis 2012;25:193–8.

114. Accurso FJ, Rowe SM, Clancy JP, et al. Effect of vx-770 in persons with cystic fibrosis and the g551d-cftr mutation. N Engl J Med 2010;363:1991–2003.

115. Falkinham JO 3rd. Nontuberculous mycobacteria from household plumbing of patients with nontuberculous mycobacteria disease. Emerg Infect Dis 2011;17:419–24.

116. Thomson R, Tolson C, Carter R, et al. Isolation of nontuberculous mycobacteria (NTM) from household water and shower aerosols in patients with pulmonary disease caused by NTM. J Clin Microbiol 2013;51:3006–11.

117. Feazel LM, Baumgartner LK, Peterson KL, et al. Opportunistic pathogens enriched in showerhead biofilms. Proc Natl Acad Sci U S A 2009;106: 16393–9.

118. Ballarino GJ, Olivier KN, Claypool RJ, et al. Pulmonary nontuberculous mycobacterial infections: antibiotic treatment and associated costs. Respir Med 2009;103:1448–55.

119. Rowe SM, Borowitz DS, Burns JL, et al. Progress in cystic fibrosis and the cf therapeutics development network. Thorax 2012;67:882–90.

Surgical Approach to Pulmonary Nontuberculous Mycobacterial Infections

John D. Mitchell, MD

KEYWORDS

- Bronchiectasis • Thoracoscopic lobectomy • VATS lobectomy • Thoracoscopic segmentectomy
- VATS segmentectomy • Pneumonectomy • Lobectomy • Nontuberculous mycobacteria

KEY POINTS

- Failure of medical therapy and symptom relief are the two main indications for surgical resection in pulmonary NTM disease.
- Most indicated resections may be performed through a minimally invasive (VATS) approach.
- In general, these resections are associated with low morbidity and mortality, although more extensive resections carry higher risk.
- Although outcomes in observational studies seem promising, much more data are needed to confirm the benefits of resection in this population.

INTRODUCTION

Although the true numbers are unknown, it is generally accepted that the incidence of pulmonary nontuberculous mycobacterial (NTM) disease is increasing in North America. Although targeted antimicrobial therapy remains the mainstay of therapy in these patients, failure of medical therapy is not uncommon. The addition of adjunctive surgical resection has been suggested to improve treatment success rates in those with focal parenchymal damage, such as bronchiectasis or cavitary lung disease. The rationale for adding surgery to the treatment of affected patients is that these areas of parenchymal disease are poorly penetrated by the antibiotic therapy, and thus serve as a "reservoir" for organisms to trigger recurrent infection. In this article, the common indications, techniques, and outcomes of pulmonary NTM surgery are discussed.

INDICATIONS FOR SURGERY

All patients must meet the criteria for pulmonary NTM infection described in the recent American Thoracic Society guidelines,[1] have focal parenchymal disease amenable to resection, and possess adequate pulmonary reserve in light of the planned surgical procedure.

Three main indications for surgery exist. In most cases, resectional surgery is performed after failure of medical therapy, as a means to induce treatment success. In these cases, the parenchymal disease should be truly "focal" in nature, whereby following resection the remaining lung is relatively free of structural damage. The presence of macrolide or other significant drug resistance is an additional impetus for the consideration of surgery in this setting, because eradication of the infection with standard medical regimens becomes less likely. Although patients often view the addition

Disclosures: The author has no disclosures.

Section of General Thoracic Surgery, Division of Cardiothoracic Surgery, University of Colorado School of Medicine, C-310, 12631 East 17th Avenue, Aurora, CO 80045, USA

E-mail address: john.mitchell@ucdenver.edu

Clin Chest Med 36 (2015) 117–122

http://dx.doi.org/10.1016/j.ccm.2014.11.004

of surgery in this setting as the curative element of their therapy, it must be emphasized that the medical treatment remains the central component of their care.

The second indication for surgery in patients with NTM disease is symptom relief. Typically, these symptoms are not life-threatening (eg, intractable cough), but are bothersome and interfere with the activities of everyday life. For a few, the symptoms may relate to a potentially lethal process (eg, significant hemoptysis) that requires surgical resection to resolve permanently. It is not uncommon for patients to suffer failure of medical therapy and intractable symptoms, for which resection may be quite helpful. In cases where symptom control is the primary objective, it is understood and accepted that areas of parenchymal damage may remain following resection, although it is critical that clinicians identify and target the relevant areas producing the symptoms.

The third indication for surgery, used selectively, is to limit or slow down the progression of disease. The goal in this situation is not to eradicate the infection, but to stabilize the clinical situation and perhaps improve the effectiveness of the medical therapy. In these cases, a "debulking" of the worst areas of parenchymal damage is performed, which if left alone may accelerate or contribute to disease in previously healthy areas. An example of this approach is the patient with bilateral parenchymal disease, but with one side much more involved, largely destroyed with cavitary disease related to the NTM infection. Resection of the destroyed lung may limit the spillage (soilage) of infected secretions to the better remaining lung, and thus slow the progression of disease.

PREOPERATIVE EVALUATION

The consideration of surgery for patients with bronchiectasis and/or cavitary lung disease related to NTM infection should be discussed in a multidisciplinary setting. Only a small proportion of all patients with pulmonary NTM disease will likely benefit from the addition of surgery to their treatment regimen. At our institution, a multidisciplinary conference is held weekly and is attended by surgeons, pulmonologists, and infectious disease clinicians with specialization in respiratory infectious disease. Case histories are individually discussed, with treatment alternatives and the optimal surgical approach explored. Using this method, we believe the benefits for our patient population are maximized.

Preoperative evaluation involves an extensive assessment including radiologic and physiologic testing and sputum analysis to optimize medical

therapy. High-resolution computed tomography of the chest is performed to assess the extent of the parenchymal lung disease (**Fig. 1**). Adequate pulmonary reserve is ensured through the use of pulmonary function testing, with occasional use of perfusion scanning and exercise testing when appropriate. Cardiac evaluation may involve echocardiography to evaluate possible valvular pathology and the presence (if any) of pulmonary hypertension, and selective use of stress testing to assess coronary disease.

Bronchoscopy is performed when appropriate, primarily for diagnostic purposes and to rule out concomitant endobronchial pathology. In the setting of active hemoptysis, bronchoscopy is used to localize the source within the bronchial tree to the segmental or even subsegmental level. Collection of sputum and bronchoalveolar lavage specimens allows identification of the likely microbial pathogens. Confirmation of the presence of NTM disease was made in accordance with the guidelines published by the American Thoracic Society.[1] Evaluation of culture results includes in vitro susceptibility testing appropriate for the cultured organism.

A complete nutritional assessment is made at the time of initial presentation, and dietary supplementation is initiated when indicated. Routine use of feeding tubes is discouraged, and is likely unnecessary in those with focal disease. In select patients with significant parenchymal (typically cavitary) disease and subsequent malnutrition, placement of a percutaneous gastrostomy tube may be helpful, although even with intensive supplementation substantial weight gain is unlikely. In addition, all patients were evaluated for the presence of significant gastroesophageal reflux.

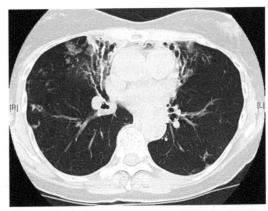

Fig. 1. Computed tomography image of a patient with NTM infection associated with right middle lobe and lingular disease, the so-called "Lady Windermere syndrome."

If present and believed to be a contributing factor to the patient's chronic pulmonary disease, recommendations are made for possible antireflux surgery with or soon after pulmonary resection.

Optimal medical therapy for patients with NTM disease is described elsewhere in this issue. Most frequently, a three- or four-drug oral antimicrobial therapy is initiated, often combined with intravenous antibiotics as indicated. Revisions to the planned therapy are occasionally made because of intolerance to the initial regimen. The duration of the preoperative antibiotic therapy varies, but typically lasts 8 to 12 weeks. The goal with the preoperative therapy is to achieve a "nadir" in the bacterial counts before surgical resection.

After the planned duration of preoperative antibiotic therapy, patients return for repeat clinical and radiologic evaluation before surgery. In select patients, repeat computed tomography scanning is used to judge the effects of the antimicrobial therapy, and to confirm stability of parenchymal disease in light of the planned procedure. The nutritional status is again evaluated if indicated, and suitability to move forward with surgery endorsed. Attention is given to other known or potential comorbidities and addressed as needed.

SURGICAL TECHNIQUE
Anesthetic Considerations

Surgical resection is performed with the patient under general anesthesia using a double-lumen endotracheal tube, or rarely a standard endotracheal tube with a bronchial blocker. Preoperative toilet bronchoscopy is selectively used to reduce the secretion burden in the airways. Epidural catheters are offered to all patients, and are favored in those undergoing thoracotomy. For those having video-assisted thoracoscopic surgery (VATS), epidurals are typically not used; intercostal blocks (0.25% bupivacaine) may be administered at the conclusion of the VATS case.

Patient Positioning

Positioning of the patient is standard. When VATS is planned, careful attention is paid to the flex or "break" in the table, to maximize the intercostal spaces in the ipsilateral hemithorax.

General Principles of Pulmonary Nontuberculous Mycobacterial Surgery

Surgical resection for infectious lung disease poses several technical challenges when compared with a similar procedure for thoracic malignancy. These differences are often neglected by the occasional NTM surgeon, who applies the more familiar oncologic techniques and principles during the procedure, leading to a suboptimal outcome. As with any complex surgical technique, these patients are usually best served by referral to centers with considerable experience in this infectious lung surgery. Anatomic lung resection (segmentectomy, lobectomy, pneumonectomy) is preferred to minimize postoperative complications and to ensure complete resection of the involved area.

Pleural adhesions are usually present to some degree, and in some cases can be extensive and vascular in nature (**Fig. 2**). They typically involve the affected segments of lung, but can also be scattered throughout the hemithorax. In cavitary upper lobe disease, the adhesions to the overlying parietal pleura can be significant. In fact, lobes with cavitary disease often have concomitant, adjacent pleural symphysis (obliteration of the pleural space), and care must be taken during lung mobilization to avoid spillage of infected debris within the pleural space (**Fig. 3**). The preoperative high-resolution computed tomography usually predicts the presence of dense adhesions, but frequently underestimates the amount of pleural symphysis. It is critical that the surgeon carefully examine the preoperative imaging to decide the best surgical approach. Most adhesions can be divided through a minimally invasive approach, often with improved visibility compared with thoracotomy. However, if widespread pleural obliteration is suspected, plans for open thoracotomy allow for dissection in the more favorable extrapleural plane. Indications to convert from VATS to an open approach include the perceived need for an extrapleural dissection, or because of concern regarding underlying vital structures.

The bronchial circulation in patients with infectious lung disease is almost always enlarged,

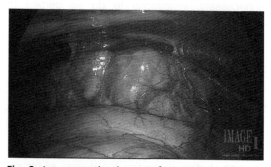

Fig. 2. Intraoperative image of a patient with right middle lobe bronchiectasis. The right lower lobe is in the foreground. Note the dense adhesions and collateral circulation present.

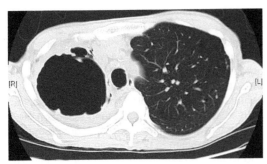

Fig. 3. Computed tomography image of a patient with severe right upper lobe cavitary disease associated with NTM infection. Complete pleural symphysis was encountered at surgery, necessitating open thoracotomy and an extrapleural dissection to minimize spillage of cavity contents within the hemithorax.

and in most cases should be addressed with clips rather than simple cautery to minimize bleeding. In addition, generalized lymphadenopathy may be present within the ipsilateral hilum. The enlarged lymph nodes may be calcified and adherent to the adjacent pulmonary vessels, making dissection difficult and hazardous. Division of lung parenchyma with staplers can also be difficult because of the chronic inflammatory process, which renders the tissue stiff, thickened, and poorly compressible.

Following segmentectomy or right middle lobe resections, a significant "residual space" is typically not an issue given the degree of parenchymal collapse or consolidation usually seen. This should be assessed on a case-by-case basis, because the residual ipsilateral lung can be poorly compliant in chronic NTM lung disease and may contribute to a space problem. In larger resections or if a significant space is anticipated, liberal use of muscle flaps, typically the latissimus dorsi, can minimize this issue.

Routine buttressing of the bronchial stump with autologous tissue to avoid bronchopleural fistula is unnecessary. Indications to do so pertain to circumstances where the risk of fistula is high: the presence of a multidrug-resistant organism, poorly controlled infection before surgery, or after right pneumonectomy.

Surgical Approach

It is possible to perform most lung resections for NTM disease in a minimally invasive fashion.[2] The key is careful examination of the preoperative imaging studies, assessing the degree of pleural symphysis. Furthermore, as surgeons gain experience in VATS approaches to infectious lung disease, mastery of the techniques used to complete the procedure safely become routine. However, if at any time the surgeon does not believe the operation cannot be done safely or in a feasible manner via VATS, conversion to open thoracotomy should be made. It is not a "complication" of the procedure to electively convert, because patient safety and correct completion of the operation trumps size of incision in all cases.

Thoracoscopic resection is done through two to four small incisions in the hemithorax, with one of the incisions enlarged to perhaps 3 cm to serve as the "access" incision from which the specimen is ultimately removed. The exact number and location of the incisions is not important, and is based on surgeon preference. Thoracoscopic or VATS procedures have two main features in common: reliance on video images to perform the case, and absence of any rib-spreading device akin to conventional thoracotomy. It is largely the latter feature that results in less pain, shorter hospital stays, and improved patient satisfaction.

Some planned resections are simply not feasible through a minimally invasive approach. Examples include cases of clear-cut pleural obliteration on the preoperative imaging studies; difficult redo anatomic resections; and most pneumonectomies, particularly those for destroyed lung. For these more complex cases, open thoracotomy provides a versatile, much safer access than a minimally invasive approach. Open thoracotomy facilitates an extrapleural dissection plane and allows for easier intrapericardial control of vessels, if needed.

Once access to the chest is obtained, resection proceeds in the same general fashion. The lung must be fully mobilized, freed of adhesions. The involved pulmonary veins and arterial branches are individually ligated, typically using stapling devices. The segmental, lobar or mainstem bronchus is isolated and also usually divided with a stapler, although hand-sewn suture closure is certainly acceptable. Careful attention to hemostasis is paramount. Closure for VATS and open cases is routine, with placement of appropriate drains.

It is important that a sample of the resected specimen be sent for culture, preferably to a laboratory with experience in mycobacterial culture techniques and testing. We routinely "double culture" all specimens, sending samples to two separate laboratories. "Culture everything" is a useful mantra, and failure to do so is illustrative of the approach of many thoracic surgeons who rarely deal with NTM disease.

Indications for muscle transposition include buttressing of the bronchial stump and to fill likely potential spaces left by the resection to minimize air leak and postoperative infectious issues. In the former case, the author prefers intercostal muscle; and in the latter, use of the latissimus dorsi muscle. In both cases, the muscle may be mobilized and transposed via either a VATS or open approach. Use of the serratus anterior muscle, although previously described, may result in winging of the scapula, which is poorly tolerated in this thin, often malnourished population.

If the patient presents for surgery with obvious contamination or soilage of the pleural space, or if it grossly occurs at operation, the surgeon must address the possibility of ongoing pleural infection. If lobectomy or less is performed, any residual pleural space can often be minimized with autologous tissue transposition, perhaps combined with thoracoplasty or transient phrenic nerve paresis. In the setting of pneumonectomy, we favor creation of an open thoracostomy (Eloesser flap) to allow packing of the space postoperatively (**Fig. 4**). Usually within several weeks to months the space is deemed ready for closure in the method of Clagett.[3]

POSTOPERATIVE CARE

In general, care of these patients, particularly after VATS resection, is routine. It is important to maintain the preoperative antibiotic regimen throughout the perioperative period. Later, as the

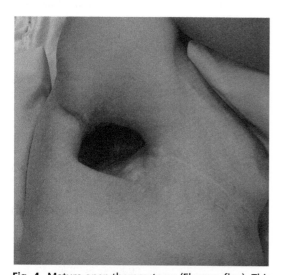

Fig. 4. Mature open thoracostomy (Eloesser flap). This patient underwent thoracotomy for blebectomy and pleurodesis as a teenager, only to return 40 years later with a destroyed right lung and gross pleural involvement associated with NTM infection. Completion pneumonectomy and open thoracostomy were performed. She underwent successful closure 1 year later.

cultures mature, modifications in the antibiotic regimen may be entertained.

COMPLICATIONS AND OUTCOMES

The outcomes of resectional surgery for pulmonary NTM disease are summarized in **Table 1**, which depicts results from the larger series in the literature.[4–9] In general, these operations, despite their complexity, may be performed with low morbidity and mortality. Some of the reported differences may be attributed to the varying patient populations and operations described. For example, outcomes of a case series concentrating on segmental resection for NTM disease is markedly different than pneumonectomy in the same population. Furthermore, it is not really appropriate to compare open and VATS procedures in terms of morbidity and mortality; the involved patient cohorts are dissimilar with respect to severity of disease and extent of operation. It is expected that VATS surgery (segmentectomy, lobectomy) in the relevant patient group (focal disease, otherwise generally healthy) will lead to less morbidity than open procedures (often pneumonectomy for severe disease) performed in malnourished individuals with multiple comorbidities. Overall, however, it seems clear that results have improved over time because of better patient selection, advances in surgical technique, postoperative care, and macrolide use.

Despite the encouraging results from the individual retrospective case series, there are very little data in the literature specifically examining the influence of surgery in patients with NTM disease. Jarand and colleagues[10] were able to demonstrate improved outcomes with the addition of surgical resection in patients with *Mycobacterium abscessus* infection. In this report of 107 patients over a 7-year period, the inclusion of surgical therapy in selected patients, compared with medical therapy alone, resulted in significantly more culture conversion and culture negativity at 1 year (57% vs 28%; $P = .022$).

CURRENT CONTROVERSIES AND FUTURE CONSIDERATIONS

Nationally, the use of surgery in this patient population remains limited, with only a few centers reporting a significant experience despite the increasing recognition of this chronic disease. This is likely caused by the paucity of comparative data demonstrating clear cut advantages to adjunctive surgical treatment, and the widespread lack of surgical expertise in this area contributing to suboptimal outcomes when surgery is

Table 1
Selected series: surgical treatment of pulmonary NTM disease

Authors,[Ref.] Year	N	Mortality (%)	Morbidity (%)	BPF (%)	Sputum Conversion (%)
Corpe,[4] 1981	131	6.9	NR	5.3	93
Nelson et al,[5] 1998	28	7.1	32	3.6	88
Watanabe et al,[6] 2006	22	0	NR	NR	95
Mitchell et al,[7] 2008	265	2.6	18.5	4.2	NR
Yu et al,[8] 2011	172	0	7	0	84
Shiraishi et al,[9] 2013	65	0	12	0	100

Abbreviation: BPF, bronchopleural fistula.

attempted. To address these issues, further research is needed studying the role of pulmonary resection in this group of patients, and thoracic surgeons need to develop a renewed focus on surgical techniques specific to infectious lung disease.

SUMMARY

The incidence of pulmonary NTM disease is increasing. Despite aggressive medical therapy, a subset of patients will experience treatment failure or suffer disabling or life-threatening symptoms. The use of anatomic lung resection in addition to optimal medical management may, in select cases, result in improved clinical outcomes. More data are needed to confirm this approach, and it is incumbent on thoracic surgeons to master the techniques needed to perform resection in those with infectious lung disease.

REFERENCES

1. Griffith DE, Aksamit T, Brown-Elliott BA, et al. An official ATS/IDSA statement: diagnosis, treatment, and prevention of nontuberculous mycobacterial diseases. Am J Respir Crit Care Med 2007;175(4):367–416.
2. Mitchell JD, Yu JA, Bishop A, et al. Thoracoscopic lobectomy and segmentectomy for infectious lung disease. Ann Thorac Surg 2012;93(4):1033–40.
3. Clagett OT, Geraci JE. A procedure for the management of postpneumonectomy empyema. J Thorac Cardiovasc Surg 1963;45(2):141–5.
4. Corpe RF. Surgical management of pulmonary disease due to *Mycobacterium avium-intracellulare*. Rev Infect Dis 1981;3(5):1064–7.
5. Nelson KG, Griffith DE, Brown BA, et al. Results of operation in *Mycobacterium avium-intracellulare* lung disease. Ann Thorac Surg 1998;66(2):325–30.
6. Watanabe M, Hasegawa N, Ishizaka A, et al. Early pulmonary resection for *Mycobacterium avium* complex lung disease treated with macrolides and quinolones. Ann Thorac Surg 2006;81(6):2026–30.
7. Mitchell JD, Bishop A, Cafaro A, et al. Anatomic lung resection for nontuberculous mycobacterial disease. Ann Thorac Surg 2008;85(6):1887–93.
8. Yu JA, Pomerantz M, Bishop A, et al. Lady Windermere revisited: treatment with thoracoscopic lobectomy/segmentectomy for right middle lobe and lingular bronchiectasis associated with non-tuberculous mycobacterial disease. Eur J Cardiothorac Surg 2011;40(3):671–5.
9. Shiraishi Y, Katsuragi N, Kita H, et al. Adjuvant surgical treatment of nontuberculous mycobacterial lung disease. Ann Thorac Surg 2013;96(1):287–91.
10. Jarand J, Levin A, Zhang L, et al. Clinical and microbiologic outcomes in patients receiving treatment for mycobacterium abscessus pulmonary disease. Clin Infect Dis 2011;52(5):565–71.

Index

Note: Page numbers of article titles are in **boldface** type.

http://dx.doi.org/10.1016/S0272-5231(15)00010-6
0272-5231/15/$ – see front matter © 2015 Elsevier Inc. All rights reserved.

Moving?

Make sure your subscription moves with you!

To notify us of your new address, find your **Clinics Account Number** (located on your mailing label above your name), and contact customer service at:

Email: journalscustomerservice-usa@elsevier.com

800-654-2452 (subscribers in the U.S. & Canada)
314-447-8871 (subscribers outside of the U.S. & Canada)

Fax number: 314-447-8029

Elsevier Health Sciences Division
Subscription Customer Service
3251 Riverport Lane
Maryland Heights, MO 63043

*To ensure uninterrupted delivery of your subscription, please notify us at least 4 weeks in advance of move.

Printed and bound by CPI Group (UK) Ltd, Croydon, CR0 4YY

03/10/2024

01040382-0005